D0594604

Susan Ager
At Heart

Editor: Helene Lorber
Illustrations: Rick Nease
Cover and book design: Karolyn Cannata-Winge

Printed in the U.S.A. on recycled paper

Detroit Free Press Inc. 1996
321 W. Lafayette Blvd.
Detroit, Michigan 48226

All rights reserved. No part of this book may be reproduced or
transmitted in any form or by any means, electronic or
mechanical, including photocopying, recording or by an
information storage system, without permission of the
publisher, except where permitted by law.

ISBN 0-937247-67-7

CONTENTS

THE MOTOR CITY

DOMESTIC RELATIONS

IN SEASON

CONVICTIONS

Foreword

Writing three columns each week is a little like going to bat three times in every baseball game of the season.

You can't expect to hit a home run each time, but that doesn't stop you from trying, from swinging too hard, from suffering when you strike out or hit a fly ball to far right field that comes this close to sailing over the fence.

I hesitate to call the columns in this book my home runs. They are, though, those that garnered lots of response, via snail mail, voice mail and — most recently — E-mail. They are ones readers I meet at the supermarket or on the street tell me they fondly remember — or wish they could forget.

Others are personal favorites, including three essays I wrote long before beginning a regular column in 1992.

I'd like to confess one insecurity: I sometimes wish I wrote "bigger" columns about, you know, issues involving the future of civilization, or matters of utmost significance to men and women with huge desks and big windows on high floors.

Instead, I tend to write about smaller matters: moments, memories, brief conversations, tickles of feeling that take us by surprise. I could argue, of course, that these things are big, because they're universal. All of us know what shame feels like, or relief, or trepidation. Most of us know the tremors of falling in love.

Thus, I write about what we share, at heart. That's where we have the most in common.

I have everyone to thank, for living your lives in my vision and within my earshot. Mostly I thank the two people who taught me to pay attention. Mom taught me sensitivity, an eye and ear for nuance. And Dad insisted I learn that there's no such thing as a stupid question.

Several editors over the years have pushed me to ask more and say more in my work, especially when I felt uneasy about my own convictions. Those editors include Patrick Connolly at the Associated Press, Iris Frost at the San Jose Mercury, and Kathy Warbelow, Brian Dickerson, Ann Olson and Steve Grimmer at the Detroit Free Press. Brian, in particular, is a good buddy, poking at my preconceptions, driving me crazy by messing up everything I've arranged so neatly in my head. And, he makes me laugh.

I owe gratitude to several people whose abiding support for my column has been notable: Laurie Hertzel, Don Kubit, Chip Visci and a certain reader I've never met, Katherine Nicholson.

My deepest gratitude goes to Larry Coppard, the man with whom I share my home, my bed and every single one of my anxieties. He speaks reason to my emotion, believes in me, and sustains me every day.

Lastly, I thank the many people who, over the years, have trusted me enough to let me tell their stories. And I thank the countless readers who have reacted, in one way or another, to my words.

They keep me in the game.

Susan Ager
Detroit, Michigan

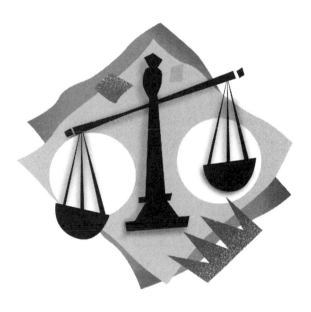

CHOICES

Moved by possibilities

At dusk, before the light of day was gone, we left our dinners half-finished on the table and drove to see a house where, that afternoon, a red-and-white sign in the yard had caught my eye: FOR SALE BY OWNER.

I've passed it hundreds of times, and admired its age, and its lines, and the young red maple that is the last in the neighborhood to burst into flaming color each fall.

We are not in the market for a house. We have settled into ours after seven years, or is it eight? But when I passed that house, whose lawn had started to turn green, whose trees were beginning to bud, I felt an unusual urgency.

After my first phone call, I told my husband, "This is the house of our dreams." After my second phone call, the owner allowed us to come by right away.

She warned us the house would smell of garlic-broccoli stir-fry, but when we stepped through the back door I noticed first three pots of miniature daffodils abloom on a wide wood windowsill.

Spring, manifest in her kitchen.

As we walked through the house, over old hardwood floors, my heart beat faster. Its walls were plaster, its woodwork a deep rich brown.

"Isn't this wonderful?" I whispered to my husband when the owner was out of earshot. "I can see why you would like it," he replied.

In the attic, the owner had built a loft, carpeting it and adding simple wood trim and a few windows. She used the space to sleep, she told us, and to meditate.

I could imagine myself moving into this house and becoming, too, a woman of serenity and strength. Buying daffodils for my sill. Drinking black coffee on spring mornings on the brick terrace right outside the kitchen door. Cutting lilacs from the huge bushes that surround the yard and piling them into old vases.

During the half-hour in which we toured the house, I changed my life. I changed myself. I changed our life together, and I invited over everyone we knew for big picnics. I imagined my nephews delighted to sleep in the loft, looking down on the park across the street where I could see us flying kites.

In our life now, we have no room or time for picnics. My nephews have never spent the night. Nor have we ever flown a kite.

I am not a woman of impulse. My father taught me to check out every appliance store in the city before buying even a toaster.

But recently two of my best friends bought houses on impulse. Walking by, falling in love, making an offer and hearing "Yes."

I am afraid to choose for fear of regrets. The only exhilaration I find in change comes years later, looking back, once things are settled again.

Which is why it felt so good to want that old house so much.

My husband and I drove home in silence, as I imagined repainting its upstairs bathroom. We sat on our sofa, at opposite ends, our legs entwined. He said, "I don't see how it would improve our life." I said, "But it has a screened-in porch, like you've always wanted!" He said, "It needs major plumbing and electrical work." I said, "How could you tell?"

"I could tell," he insisted, then said: "If you want it, call and make an offer." Having assessed, evaluated and drawn a negative conclusion, he tossed the ball to me, with only whim and desire on my side.

I poured myself a half-glass of wine. He went to his study. By 11 p.m., we had shoved the house from our minds as the obligations of our tomorrows oozed in to fill the space.

In the morning neither of us mentioned it.

But, late for work, I still drove out of my way to pass the house where, despite winter's lingering chill, sunlight flooded the brick terrace, pouring in through the window where the daffodils bloom.

April 6, 1995

The drug trip

America is growing older, and here's how we can tell: Drug use by adults is way down from the mid-1980s.

The statistics are stark: A third as many people said they used cocaine in 1991 than 1985, and half as many said they smoked marijuana.

But statistics are less meaningful than stories. Here's one from a friend, who lived it.

My friend is in his late 20s, an accomplished professional, well-regarded in his field.

Being in his 20s, he's danced a lot with drugs. Once he and a friend, headed for Jamaica and afraid of customs officials, bought a bottle of Tylenol, emptied all the capsules and refilled them with Ecstasy, the drug they thought they could not do without.

Their ruse succeeded. But that was years ago, when they were young and haughty and ruthless.

Now, older, he does not do drugs so often. Oh, his brother will occasionally roll him a joint, which he smokes to be polite. But hard drugs are rare.

Except a recent weekend when he flew east for a friend's 30th birthday party.

That friend announced in advance that he would purchase cocaine for whoever wanted it. And my friend forked over the $75 required for a gram of coke these days. At the party, he snorted about a third of it.

He didn't want to do too much. He was seeing relatives the next day, and didn't want to be up all night.

So what he didn't snort he nudged into a small glass vial and took back to his hotel room.

Packing his carry-on bag the next day for his return to Detroit, he found the vial to have grown considerably — not in size, but significance. He couldn't figure out where to put it. He was afraid it would show up on the airport bag X-ray, and that they would ask him what it was. He was afraid that if he carried it in a pocket, some belt buckle would set off the security alert, and he'd have to empty his pockets, and there would be the vial of cocaine. The vial became a terrible, frightening challenge. He imagined prison. He imagined humiliation. He imagined losing his good job, and his friends' respect. But he couldn't believe that, not yet 30, he was worried about these things! What an old man he was becoming! What an old fart!

He moved the vial four times before he reached the airport.

Once there, he thought about the $50 worth of cocaine it held. He wondered when he would use it. Certainly not in the mornings, because it would make him too jittery to do his work well. And not in the evenings, either. Because while he used to be able to stay wide awake till 5 a.m., he couldn't do that now. He had things to get done the next day: work, chores, life.

As he stood in the crowd at the airport, he felt the vial burning a hole in his clothing, and his future.

So he reached into his back pants pocket, where he had last hid it, and slipped it into a trash can.

Fifty dollars, into the trash.

Because he is older now. Successful now. Because he has a lot to lose.

And because he's smart enough to know that. I asked him how he felt afterward.

"Sad," he said. "Confined."

I knew he was talking about more than drugs. That I understood.

Still, I thought: "You'll get over it."

Most adults do.

August 12, 1993

One for the books

Gingerly, I step into John Printz's home. I turn sideways to squeeze past the front door. It opens only halfway because behind it are stacks of books. Beyond it are stacks of books. Everywhere I can see are piles of books — three, four, five feet high.

He has dropped his coat onto a nose-high pile in the vestibule, the hall closet having long ago been blocked shut by books. I drop mine there, too.

Now what? No passageways exist among the books. Instead, I hike my skirt and lift one leg very high, over cardboard boxes of Austen and Dreiser and Sagan and Elmore Leonard, dropping my shoe into what tiny space I can find.

Printz leads, teetering as he vaults from footprint to footprint. I do, too, knowing one stumble would trigger an avalanche.

"I don't move around the house much," says Printz, who is 51 and lives alone. "I only have to get into it once a day."

Ask him to diagnose his condition, and he says instantly, "Bibliomania!" then laughs with delight. He is a man who once kept his library neatly on shelves, but who over 20 years has let books engulf his furniture, his home and his life.

He says: "You are the first person in here in eight years.

"I have no friends," he adds without remorse. "I've found I can't learn anything from talking to people. People say things, but it adds up to nothing." Nor does he want friends. "They take time. And time is precious if you're trying to learn."

His last visitor was a census-taker, who asked a few quick questions and fled. "I'm not a normal person. And this," he nods at his books, "doesn't make any sense to people."

At first, it makes no sense to me, either. How can someone be so shockingly out of control? Who is this man I'm following deeper into a trap of books?

I know some people collect thousands of hubcaps, or 2,700 pairs of shoes, or hundreds of sets of salt-and-pepper shakers. But I imagine they keep their obsessions in order, in a garage or closet or one corner of their otherwise conventional lives. The only corners of John Printz's home without books are those with radiators.

Away from home, he unpacks and checks in new books for Wayne State University's libraries, a job he's had for 22 years. On Saturdays, making the rounds of Detroit's used-book stores, he buys paperbacks and hardbacks, most of them inexpensive. He spends perhaps $125 each week — or about $6,500 a year of his $32,000 salary.

"I'm interested in about 100 topics," he says, but concentrates on this odd mix: Bible history. Ancient history. Philosophy. The classics. Opera. And the history of motor-car racing.

He carries the books back to his one-bedroom house near Grand River and Greenfield and sets them down, in an order only he discerns. He reads some, or parts of some, and parts of some over and over again. Albert Schweitzer's "The Quest of the Historical Jesus" required almost 10 years' effort to comprehend, he admits. And, he has reread the Gospel of Mark at least 1,000 times, from the 300-some Bibles he owns, many in languages he doesn't know.

For relief, he reads modern fiction — Hammett, Chandler, LeCarre — and nearly anything else he hears people talking about, although he's often disappointed.

He reads in an old wooden office chair in the kitchen, although he must first clear its lap of books. Or, he reads in bed, cushioned by a single thin pillow, surrounded by a wall of books three feet high.

He can explain his mania only this way: Books offer knowledge, for which he has always hungered. Since second grade he knew he was different. In high school, he read Spinoza, Voltaire, Gibbon, while other kids goofed off. His grades plummeted as he spun off in other directions to learn.

"When I was a kid, I realized a man of knowledge was a rarity, and I thought it would be noble to become one. But I've had to wake up to the fact that people really aren't interested in knowledge.

"So you do it for yourself. To other people, it doesn't mean anything."

He earned a degree in history from Wayne State. And, for a few years, he was married. She left in 1978, for reasons only partly to do with his books. Once she was gone, though, books took over.

They engulfed the red couch, surrounded and obscured every table, climbed up the walls like vines. In each room, the stacks along the edges are neat, but books bought more recently are mounded in the middle in misshapen cardboard boxes.

"I never used the furniture anyhow," he shrugs. "To read, I need nothing more than a chair."

He owns no TV, and eats all meals out. Books block his avocado refrigerator, which he last used about 15 years ago and which may, he guesses, still contain a beer or two brought over by a woman. He doesn't drink, never has. Books fill his kitchen sink, and all the floor space in his bathroom. The tub and sink and toilet are usable, but brown with 20 years' grime.

Cooking and cleaning take time.

The Ping-Pong table in the basement on which he used to play is sagging with thousands of books. Books teeter atop the washer, dryer and laundry tubs. The basement and attic steps are passable only if you are nimble and press your palms against the walls to keep from tumbling. Thousands more books weigh down the attic.

He likes his home, and travels only to auto races, having witnessed every Indy 500 for the past 37 years. Otherwise, he never leaves the city.

"Emerson said travel is a fool's paradise," he says. "I wouldn't go quite so far. But I know some people who go to see the Parthenon, and they come back with no idea what they looked at, or who built it. I say to them, 'Did you know the Parthenon was built with stolen money?' And they look at me kind of funny, and I say, 'You should read Thucydides on the Peloponnesian Wars,' and they're rather in a state of shock."

He's proud of what he's learned, and at what a bargain. "The universe is all here," he says, raising his bushy eyebrows in wonder. "Anything that's known has been recorded in a book, so you've got the whole world at your feet."

But standing in a footprint in his kitchen, with no place to sit or even lean, he seems a lonely man, isolated by a moat filled with old words by dead men on dry pages.

When I ask him about regrets, he seems flustered by my failure to understand.

"I am gainfully employed. I have had the same job for 22 years. I do not get angry. I do not get depressed. And I would not trade places with anyone else in the world.

"I have only one desire: to know more."

I think: If John Printz had money and privilege, perhaps he would hire someone to keep his obsession in order, to build more bookcases, to add a wing to the house, to make people like me feel more at ease. Instead, Printz spends all his time and all his money buying what he loves, wallowing in it, and to hell with control.

So his books pile up. So what? So far, they have not crushed him.

As the evening winds down, Printz does not push me out. He will talk for hours, if I'd like to listen, about all that he knows.

When I leave, he leads me cautiously to the door. He steps into the cold on the porch to give me room to put on my coat. Then I squeeze out and into the vast world again, where almost everybody keeps tight control of their timid hungers, while he steps back inside with his books.

February 17, 1993

Midday, at 40

Coasting toward my 40th birthday as if it were any old birthday, I heard a few words on the radio that startled me.

I was half-listening to National Public Radio when a man mentioned the birth of a baby — "a baby," he said, "at the dawn of its day."

The face behind my face frowned, and the voice inside my head said, "If a baby is at the dawn of its day, where — at 40 — am I?"

I am at 2 o'clock in the afternoon, I decided. Or 3. Or maybe even 4.

The light is changing in my life. Although several hours of good sunlight remain, and the evening holds its own allure, my morning is gone.

High noon passed and I didn't even notice.

The metaphor stunned me and tears came to my eyes: I'm in midafternoon of my day, my only day.

Did I spend too long in my pajamas?

I've blown my share of moments in this, my only day, by being fearful, petulant or childish. I tend to expect a whole lot of everything, then mope when I'm disappointed.

I'm ashamed to say I've stained any number of anniversary and birthday celebrations wishing, for example, that I had a poet for a husband instead of a man who loves me with unembellished reliability, day after day.

But in my midafternoon now, geez! There's no time for dawdling, for sighing, for excuses.

You can spend a lifetime scanning your sky and the shifting clouds of your personality, Susan, putting off action for the sake of analysis. Or you can accept that you're complex and baffling, just like everybody else, and get on with it.

You can spend too many calories on angst, with all the rules of life you've learned rattling around in your head, bouncing up against each other, making you feel that you're doing everything wrong. Living wrong. Making wrong choices. Or, for fear of wrong choices, making no choices at all.

Interesting: Oprah turned 40 a few days ago, model Christie Brinkley turned 40 yesterday and I turn 40 tomorrow. I considered feeling terrible that one is rich and one is gorgeous and I am neither. Then I decided to quit competing with the whole damned world and recognize, with some awe and humility, that we each spend our days differently, and that the only day I have to play out is my own.

Does everybody turning 40 speak in such cliches? I guess experience feels like wisdom to us, but must amuse everyone who's older. They've discarded these cliches long ago for new ones.

The bottom line is there's no making sense of growing older, so you do a little turning-40-50-60 dance, restyling yourself, redefining the purpose of your life, so you don't dwell too much on the sad, hard truth: You've lost the high hope of morning and the excitement of a vast day ahead of you.

This weekend we're visiting my mother-in-law, who happens to have turned 80 two days ago. I don't think I'll tell her my metaphor about the day. She would laugh and roll her eyes, amused at my melodrama, and say, "I guess that means I'm on the brink of midnight," as if midnight were any old hour.

February 3, 1994

A plan for death

Our friend Phil is dying of brain cancer, but too slowly.
Weeks ago when we visited, he repeated to us several times from the hospital bed in his Chicago apartment, "I'm ready to die." When we held his limp hand, and kissed his face good-bye, we thought he might go that evening.

But days and nights passed. "I want to die," he says, over and over. Yet death is dawdling. Now Phil is on morphine. Just days ago, his doctor put him on Prozac, too — to help him put on a happy face, I guess, during his anguishing last days.

On Monday he couldn't get a single word out. For six hours, on and off, dozing and waking, he struggled to voice the word. His wife thought it was something he wanted to eat. Finally, bingo! Listening closely, she heard him say "chair." He wanted to be lifted from his bed on a special sling and lowered into his recliner by the window.

Phil is 52. He never made plans for this kind of death. For years he knew he was sick, but thought he could beat it. Once he conceded that he wouldn't, he figured death would be swift. Now it's too late: Phil never asked anyone to help hasten his death, and now he can't ask and none of us dare intervene.

Meanwhile, in a Livonia nursing home, my 84-year-old grandmother wears diapers 24 hours a day and won't leave her room. Her food is ground to a mush. She is confused by Alzheimer's disease, but when my parents visit she typically greets them with this question: "Are you here to help me die?"

She's on Prozac, too.

In her room she is the youngest. In the middle bed lies a 94-year-old woman, an incessant babbler. And next to her is a 104-year-old woman who sits silently in her wheelchair, her eyes squinched shut, her mouth working as if a piece of food is caught in her teeth, now and again shrieking, "Help me! Help me!"

No one pays attention. Calls for help are background noise here.

It's too late for these women. If ever they planned a way out of their lives, they let pass the last moment when they had the strength and wits to achieve it. In their final days, they're trapped.

Meanwhile, Jack Kevorkian rejects breakfast in jail. The Michigan Court of Appeals considers legal questions that are higher on its stack than the assisted suicide law. Months will pass before Kevorkian comes to trial. Years will pass, surely, before society figures out how to regulate induced death.

Which is why some young and healthy people I know, including me, already are making plans. Buying guidebooks like "Final Exit." Wringing promises from friends, relatives, doctors to help them die when the time comes, even though their hearts might break to do so. The wisest collect pledges from a half dozen people so that when the going gets tough, at least one can be counted on to come through.

In the end, the woman with the best-laid plans still might decide she'd rather wait for death's own pace. A man might conclude the sight of snow from his window is enough to live for. Anyone might lapse into a coma or incoherence before being able to signal for death to the most committed helpmate.

But without any plans at all, they have no hope for escape.

December 2, 1993

A fine Polish name

When he was born 32 years ago, his mother named him Joseph Conrad, after the Polish-born novelist, which would have been swell except that he also acquired his father's surname.

Joseph Conrad Mikolajczyk grew up with a name strangers pronounced correctly one of 100 times, if that.

Each September morning when a new teacher called attendance, Joe waited for his name to be mangled. He learned to anticipate the moment when his turn would come, and the instant he heard the teacher say "Joe" he'd shoot his hand into the air and yelp "Here!"

Correct Polish pronunciation of the name is mee-koh-WHY-check, but the family concluded early that most Americans would not swallow that. So each time they checked in with a restaurant hostess, or left film at a drugstore for processing, or ordered a pizza, they substituted an easier name: Michaels.

Joe and his five siblings grew up unintimidated by long complicated words. Often they starred in spelling bees.

His brother Tim, 10 years older than Joe, got a special kick from his last name. "Take your time," he'd tell strangers struggling to sound it out. "Give it your best shot." He loved it when an old Pole smiled in recognition. And he liked to quote a line he heard his dad use: "It's a hard name to pronounce, but I'm an easy guy to get along with."

He even dumped girlfriends who would tease him about the name and vow, if they ever married, to keep their own.

Joe was equally proud of his name but realized as he grew up in Redford that it baffled most people. In high school he modified the pronunciation to mi-kohl-EYE-chick, but that didn't help much. Finally, after he got his MBA and a job as public relations director for the Michigan Cancer Foundation, someone mispronounced it Michael-Isaac, and Joe pounced on that as his best pronunciation bet:

Familiar words. Familiar sounds. Easy to remember.

His wife, Rebecca, though, stuck to mi-kohl-EYE-chick. She hadn't hesitated to assume his 11-letter last name. Women do it all the time: You love a man, you take his name. But in her law firm, she is the only person paged by first name only. And her boss, with whom she has worked for four years, still hesitates to introduce her.

"People are afraid they'll embarrass you by screwing it up, or embarrass themselves by sounding ignorant," she says.

Joe admits a name like that comes in handy as a screening device when the phone rings in the evening. Callers who stumble over it obviously don't know him well enough to be interrupting his dinner.

Joe's sisters married out of the name, one becoming a Jennings, the other a Jurkiewicz, which everyone had to admit is only marginally easier than Mikolajczyk.

And Joe and his older brother John began thinking of escaping the name, too. Of legally changing it to Michaels, which had served them in public places for years. It would, they thought, make a fine and simple new name, especially for their young children, set to enter school systems not run by Polish nuns.

Everybody they told about it had a black or white opinion, and Joe agonized. The name is centuries old, and served other men well. But it's only a name. He felt proud of his heritage, and lived by many Polish traditions, but wanted non-Poles to feel more at ease with him. He wanted a name people could speak without stammering. And he wanted his kids to have an easier time than he did.

He wanted their names to fit in the boxes on application forms.

His sister, the one who became a Jennings, gave Joe grief about it.

"You're one to talk!" he scoffed.

"Joe," she replied, "we're talking life here, not Little Caesars."

Joe and John worried, too, about their father's reaction. He had been a Mikolajczyk longer than any of them. They knew that once, when he was young, he had planned to shorten his name until his mother, an immigrant, had protested. "Why?" she had asked him. "Are you ashamed of your name?"

But she was long dead, and Dad wasn't sentimental. He gave Joe and John his blessing. And that made all the difference.

"My father is the most important role model in my life," Joe said. "If he didn't approve, I wouldn't have thought again about it."

Weeks before Joe and John went to court to finalize the change, Joe broke the news to his 3½-year-old son, who has been able to pronounce his name since he was 2. Little Daniel asked the same question: "Why, Daddy? I like my name." Joe groaned and wondered again if he was doing the right thing.

Last Wednesday, in front of a clerk at the Wayne County Probate Court, and at a cost of about $100, the deed was quickly done, without emotion or ceremony, as routinely as the 1,200 other name changes that pass through the court each year.

Joseph Conrad Mikolajczyk became Joseph Conrad Michaels. His brother John's name changed, too, and their wives' names, and their children's names.

Notes will be attached to their birth certificates. It's up to them to change everything else: business cards, voice mail greetings, credit cards, bank accounts, Social Security records, driver's licenses, car and voter registrations, and the brass engraved knocker that hangs on Joe's front door.

All that takes only time. Harder will be growing accustomed to thinking of themselves by names they've seen only on pizza boxes.

In the days after the change, Joe said: "It's OK to be proud of your heritage, but a last name is only a last name. I want people to know and respect me for who I am, not for my last name."

His brother Tim said: "My name is like a limb or something. I would never get rid of it. I tell my own son to remember that his name is unique, just like him. I love my brothers and will love them forever. But I'd just as soon stay the way I am."

As for the novelist Joseph Conrad, he was christened Josef Teodor Konrad Walecz Korzeniowski. And changed his name, too.

April 10, 1994

Sober strangers can't think clearly

At midnight after a fancy event in downtown Detroit, I found myself in a valet line behind a middle-aged man who seemed very drunk.

"Ah! My good friend!" he shouted as I approached. I vaguely recalled shaking his hand early in the evening, but couldn't remember his name or anything else about him except that he was sober then.

Several of us were waiting for our cars, hunched in a chill wind, most of us alone, none of us friends.

But the drunk man united us into an uneasy audience.

"I'm not sure I can find my way home tonight!" he exclaimed, as if proud of himself. His eyes were red and he swayed a little.

"Uh-oh," someone said. Someone else asked, "How far do you have to go?"

"About 60 miles," he beamed, naming a northern suburb.

Murmurs.

"You should call a cab," someone said firmly. "We should call a cab for you," someone else said tentatively.

"Oh no, no, no," he insisted. "I'll be fine."

The valet was delivering my car. I got into it just as another valet delivered his.

On my way home, I thought about him, meandering alone on the freeway after midnight.

"Take the keys, call a cab," the ads say. "Friends don't let friends drive drunk."

But this guy wasn't a friend. None of us knew him. We were tired. Our feet hurt. We wanted to get home. Perhaps he wasn't as drunk as he seemed.

So we let him go.

The next morning, I felt troubled. Part of me wanted to forget it. Chances were he got home fine. And if he hadn't, I'd likely never hear whom he hurt or killed. But I knew we — or I — ought to have done something.

My husband agreed: "You should have grabbed his keys and thrown them in the river."

Then he told me a story:

Many years ago, he trailed a drunk driver for a few miles one night. Finally, at a stoplight, my husband rushed out of his car, yanked open the drunk's passenger door, reached in and pulled the keys from the ignition, tossing them over his shoulder. Then he jumped in his car and drove away.

He presumes the man found a pay phone and a ride home. Or the cops found him stranded in the intersection. All my husband cared about was that he no longer was piloting a 3,000-pound machine.

I was dumbfounded. I couldn't imagine caring enough or daring enough to do such a thing. I asked: "Didn't you feel like a bully?"

"Not at all. He was a drunk!"

"What if he'd had a gun?"

"We didn't worry about that in those days."

The executive director of Michigan's MADD chapter had better ideas. Bethany Goodman suggested someone from our group in line ought to have alerted a valet who might have withheld the man's keys and called a cab.

"Might" is the key word. Lawyers say the establishment that served him too many drinks is clearly legally liable. But a valet who lets him drive away likely has no more legal obligation to stop him than those of us at the curb.

Goodman had another idea: Any of us with a car phone should have dialed 911 to warn the cops about a motorist wandering I-75 in a haze.

Her suggestions seemed so obvious I felt ashamed for not having thought of them on the spot.

I guess it was late. I guess I was tired. I guess we all were.

At high noon any of us would agree that stopping a drunken driver is the right thing to do, that we stand morally liable. But sadly, at midnight in the '90s, it's easier to turn away and just go home.

May 10, 1993

A smaller sip of wine

My name is Susan, and I am not an alcoholic.
Nor am I powerless.

I had a problem with alcohol — I drank it every night.

But I no longer do, thanks to one of the new moderation programs that helped me tame what had become a bad habit.

I'm confident I won't drink every night anymore, or let my alcohol habit control me. Still, I'm glad I can enjoy a fine glass of merlot now and again or a smoky single-malt scotch — by choice, not compulsion.

Am I in denial? I don't think so. I never denied I had a problem. My problem was this: I would wake up most mornings a little foggy and think: "I'm too old to be drinking two or three glasses of wine each night. Tonight, no wine for me."

But by nightfall my resolve had faded. Driving home from work I would imagine the whole wine-drinking ritual: uncorking the bottle, pouring it into my favorite glass, sipping it while I made dinner. On most nights, I was drinking before I even opened the mail.

The next morning I made a new resolution to do without wine. I resolved 100 times, 200 times, to break the nightly habit. I failed just as many times.

Did I get slobbering drunk? Never. Did I miss work? Never. Did I hide bottles? Never. Did I black out or drive drunk or suffer debilitating hangovers?

Never.

But did I buy three or four bottles of wine per week? Yes. Week after week? Yes. Was there always wine in the house? Sure. Would I go out into a thunderstorm for a bottle? I never had to. I planned ahead.

Did I drink alone? You bet. It was among my favorite pastimes: Coming home to an empty house, opening a new bottle, then sitting by candlelight with my food and my wine and my book and reading and drinking.

Most nights I faded off into sleep, having accomplished very little.

The next evening I found I had to reread what I had read the night before.

At dinner parties, wine turned the conversation scintillating. But why couldn't I remember the details the next day? It seemed so fascinating the night before, insights and witticisms I'd never forget.

I knew I was in real trouble, though, when my evenings were consumed by other things, but I still needed a drink to sleep. One night we drove for many hours, but when we reached our motel at midnight I said, "Let's go out for a scotch." I had fantasized about it for hundreds of miles.

I didn't always drink this way. In college I hated beer — still do. I remember drinking over a four-year period the occasional blackberry brandy, two or three Singapore Slings and a glass or two of Cold Duck on New Year's Eve.

My first post-college boyfriend and I drank rum-and-Tabs now and again in bed, and another boyfriend and I liked sipping brandy on the roof of my apartment at midnight.

I did not drink nightly until a few years ago, when I began writing this column. I felt nervous and anxious and afraid: of failure, of criticism, and of who I was, naked and revealed by the column.

With every column I tried to hit a home run, but of course many of my swings resulted in limp grounders. I came home every night with a thousand voices in my head: readers, editors, coworkers, family members and my own crew of internal critics.

To quiet the voices, I would pour myself a glass of wine.

Soon, one glass didn't shut off the noise. Two worked better.

Anyone who drinks knows that your body builds a tolerance to alcohol.

Two won't give you the buzz one used to. You spill a bit more into your glass. Two becomes three. On bad nights, three becomes four. Soon you are drinking most of a bottle of wine and thinking: "This has got to stop."

I cried out for help for eight months before taking real action. I confided in friends who are recovering alcoholics who said, yes indeed, I had a problem and suggested I consult Alcoholics Anonymous. I spoke with doctors and nurses who disagreed, who said two or three glasses each night was OK. I read articles that said a woman who drinks two glasses of wine each night decreases her risk of a heart attack but increases her risk of breast cancer.

Despite the mixed messages, I knew I had to stop. It scared me that I couldn't break my habit with sheer willpower. Turns out I just didn't know how.

I found in a newspaper a tiny ad that caught my eye: "DrinkWise: Healthy choices for people who drink."

I cut it out. A few days later, I called for information. They sent it to me, and I read it in bed one night as I sipped from the wineglass almost always at my bedside. The problem drinker it described sounded a lot like me.

But six months passed. I didn't want to spend hundreds of dollars to get help I thought I could give myself for free.

In those six months I vowed to quit many more times. I drank another 100 bottles of wine. I began to feel ashamed each week when I pulled my recycling bin out to the curb.

Two last straws fell on my heap: First, I read a memoir by writer and newspaper columnist Pete Hamill called "A Drinking Life." I chose it deliberately, thinking it would scare me into solving my problem.

He drank for decades, and much more than I ever did, but quit cold turkey one New Year's Eve after realizing his life had become scripted, not spontaneous. His memory — any writer's best tool — was continually fogged by alcohol. After he quit he soon realized, "I'd been squeezing my talent out of a toothpaste tube. I'd misused it and abused it and failed to replenish it with deep reading and full consciousness."

Then, at my stepson's wedding, I sat next to his bride's father, a recovering alcoholic for 10 years. As we talked about his past, he sounded strong and in control, and I, two or three wines into the evening, sounded fuzzy and vulnerable.

Later that evening, when my brother-in-law suggested we stop by a jazz club for a bedtime scotch, I did not know how to say no, and went along, and drank that scotch, all the while wondering what was wrong with me.

The next morning I said out loud to my husband: "I do not want to awaken each morning of the rest of my life disappointed in myself."

I called DrinkWise at the University of Michigan Medical Center and made an appointment.

My counselor, Nancy Holmes, made it clear at our first session that the program wasn't for everyone. "When is the last time you consumed 10 drinks on one occasion?" she asked, and I gasped. People who regularly drink that much probably had a physical dependence on alcohol that moderation could not temper.

She told me a third of Americans don't drink at all, and that of those who drink, most do so moderately and socially. A small percentage are alcoholics, able to save themselves only through abstinence.

But many problem drinkers like me can learn ways to cut back, by analyzing why and when we drink and devising and practicing new behaviors, including words to say to ourselves and others. Keeping track of how much you drink also helps, just like tracking fat grams in your diet, so I began jotting on my calendar each night how many drinks I had that day.

She asked me what I thought triggered my drinking: Certain friends? Certain situations? Without hesitation I said, "Evening. Evening triggers my drinking." I sighed. She smiled. Even that habit, she said, can be broken.

The first week of the eight-week program, I cut back to one glass of wine each night — a very distinct change made worse because a mere glass could no longer soothe me. I said glumly to my husband: "This is like drinking Kool-Aid. There's no point."

Nancy asked me to go completely free of alcohol for the next two weeks.

We made an exception for Thanksgiving and decided on that day I would have one glass of wine in midafternoon and one with dinner. I learned that thinking ahead, deciding how to drink and rehearsing ways to succeed helped a lot.

But the night before Thanksgiving posed my first and biggest challenge. We arrived at our good friends' home late, after a long drive. We stepped through the back door and our host Bob strolled into the kitchen to welcome us.

He held a drink in his hand, a fragrant single-malt scotch. I could smell it. I could hear the tinkle of ice. And I could imagine the ease it gave him.

"Can I get you a scotch?" he said, and I summoned all the strength of will I had to speak one of my practiced lines: "No, thanks. I'm cutting back."

My habit urged me to say yes, but my training helped me to say no.

While my husband and our friends drank scotch that night, I

sipped soda water with lime. Funny, once I had a glass in my hand and something to sip, I felt fine. Strong. Even a little smug.

In the three months since I began to tame my drinking, my weekly consumption has fallen from about 20 drinks to about three or four, spread over two or three evenings. Most nights I write a big fat 0 in my date book.

I tell myself: "I don't need a drink tonight." Instead, I pour into my old favorite wineglass some low-cal cranberry juice and soda water. When I'm upset or hurt, I remind myself: "You shouldn't drink to cope." A hot cup of Lemon Zinger tea calms me now.

When I drink to be festive, one glass of wine gives me the buzz that three failed to do before. I savor wine now, and enjoy it more.

I calculate that about 200 glasses of wine have gone unconsumed by me since I started the program. That's about 33 bottles.

I've lost about 13 pounds and counting, passing up 30,000 wine calories and snacking less in the evening.

In the morning I feel brighter. I need less coffee. My complexion and my brain are clearer. My face is less puffy, my nose less often red. Mostly, I like myself more. I feel in control again.

I wish I had been able to curb my drinking on my own, the way many people do as they grow older and wiser. Instead, I needed structure and guidelines and goals.

I also wish critics of moderation programs like the one I joined understood them better. DrinkWise would never suggest that everyone can have a few drinks. Some people cannot. AA has saved many of those people, and they dare not touch alcohol again for fear of falling back into an abyss.

Why scoff at folks like me who found salvation somewhere else, by different rules? Even a good friend of mine, an AA veteran, told me he thinks I am fooling myself.

I don't think I am. Just as not every sick person needs open-heart surgery, not every drinker needs abstinence.

I'm glad I found DrinkWise. It saved me for the second half of my life.

Call DrinkWise in Ann Arbor at 1-313-747-9473 anytime. Or access it on the Internet at **http:/www.med.umich.edu/drinkwise**.

February 4, 1996

Wanted: Life coach

Choked by smoke and fear, the 50,000 people who evacuated the World Trade Center after a deadly explosion had no choice but to get out the best they could.

No one stood in the stairwell with a loudspeaker, giving directions. No one broadcast instructions over the PA system, as if in an exercise video. No workers carried in their wallets little cards detailing evacuation procedures.

A lucky few carried flashlights. The rest had nothing but their wits.

One woman, after emerging safe and sound, whined to interviewers: "Nobody was there to tell us what to do."

"Yeah, lady," I said out loud to my TV. "Whaddaya expect?!? This is life."

Nobody's ever there to tell you what to do when you really need it: When your kid is crying because nobody likes him. When someone you love hears a terminal diagnosis. When you learn you've been betrayed. When you find a thousand-dollar bill lying on the sidewalk. When a fire destroys the memories of a lifetime, or a bomb explodes in your building.

What do I do first? What do I do next? What do I say? What do I skip? When do I stop?

Eventually I cooled down at the whiny woman on TV because I, too, have felt as she did. Sometimes, when I'm utterly overwhelmed, I wail to my husband, "I just want someone to run my life for me!"

I envy Olympic athletes — not for their bodies, but for their coaches. Off camera, day after day, coaches advise and guide. On camera, at the sidelines, they whisper things in athletes' ears. They watch, they nod, they frown. Sometimes a coach even weeps with joy at an athlete's achievement and wraps the athlete in a tremendous hug.

Those scenes bring tears to my eyes. They make me think, "Well, damn! If I had a full-time coach, I could do great things, too."

What I long for is a "life coach" — someone small enough to fit in my pocket, whom I could carry wherever I go. My coach would kick me in the ass when I needed it, cheer me on when I succeeded and console me when I failed. My coach would know when to hold my hand and when to prick my billowing ego. My coach would amplify the whimper of my conscience and muzzle the shouts of my fears.

My coach would tell me what to do, and I would trust my coach to be right.

When I was little, I had an invisible coach. I called her my Guardian Angel. All us Catholic kids had one. Our angels were curly-haired and sweet-faced, as pictured in our catechisms, and often wore flowing blue gowns.

They had two jobs: To protect us. And to advise us.

With angels on our shoulders, we did not suffer the full fear children might be expected to feel venturing into a vast world alone. And we knew that when something scary or confusing happened, we could count on wisdom greater than our own to tell us what to do.

What a crafty educational tool, the Guardian Angel! We learned to trust that voice in our heads, believing it was inspired. Only later did we realize it was our own voice, all that we'd ever have.

But it's not enough. We still want someone smarter, with quick tips and snappy step-by-step instructions to get us through the real challenges of our lives — those that test our morality, our maturity, our compassion, our stamina, our resolve.

Instead, life seems a long, dark, smoky stairwell, in which we're all packed together, with no clue what to do next. Except this: To listen to the voices in our heads that say, "Keep going."

March 3, 1993

Back to the garden

Our lives are so rarely our own. But we can choose our food.
I'm back to beans.

I was a vegetarian once before, in 1974, when a nasty chemical
called PBB was accidentally mixed with livestock feed,
contaminating animals throughout the Midwest.

Petrified of weird cancers, I gave up meat, fowl, milk. I made
lentil-cheese loaves, spinach lasagna. And huge, lush salads.

Then I fell in love. Men tend to change us, and that man coaxed
me back to meat. Specifically, hamburgers.

I didn't think about vegetarianism again until I invited a long-
lost friend for dinner. I prepared for her a chicken stir-fry, which she
ate slowly and thoughtfully.

The next day she revealed by phone that she had been a
vegetarian for years, and my chicken had made her sick. She also
told me this: When she gave up meat, her bowel movements didn't
smell so bad.

Funny how you can't forget a line like that.

A few years later, I wrote about a chicken-killing contest in
northern Michigan at which 120 free-range chickens were
slaughtered by a team of 20 friends. I participated, plucking wet
feathers from warm bodies, scooping out innards with my bare
hand, smiling but sick at heart.

Then the final straw fell: My family, gathered for a summer week
on Lake Huron, fished for our lunch at a trout farm.

We needed nine, and caught them within 10 minutes. I caught
one myself. Easy.

But as I lifted it from the water, the fish twitched on the hook just
like the dying, headless chickens had flapped on the clothesline
where they were hung, upside down, to drain their blood.

The old woman who cleaned the fish pulled each one, gasping, from a bucket. She held the fish down with one hand and with the other smacked its head two or three times with a heavy club.

My dad, watching her work, remarked, "That's how they kill baby seals!"

She beat the life from those fish, then removed all the inner parts that had kept them alive.

Minutes later, my brother stuck some lemon slices where their guts used to be, grilled them with his wife's herb butter, and we ate them for lunch. Everyone said they were terrific.

I could barely swallow.

Months later I quit meat and fish altogether. It's been over a year now, and I've been seduced only three times: by a bratwurst, a slice of corned beef, and a Christmas Eve salmon filet. I'm more pragmatic than principled. I'll eat restaurant soups made with meat broth, shoving the meat chunks aside.

Otherwise I eat vegetables and beans and pastas, and am content.

Do my lapses compromise me? By strict vegetarian standards, of course. But I'm trying. I'm changing. I think more about what goes on my plate.

Life around us is so violent that to try to nourish ourselves without having caused any creature to flail and scream seems a small and honest goal.

Farming is gentle. Seeds are scattered. Rain falls. The sun sprays light on the earth. The tug that yields an ear of corn, or a tomato, or a bunch of grapes is quiet. No blood falls. There is no sign of anguish.

In my wallet I carry this quote from playwright William Saroyan: "In the time of your life, live, so that in that good time there shall be no ugliness for yourself or for any life your life touches."

I wish. I violate this daily. But every simple dinner — corn, beans, red pepper sauteed in a pan — reminds me that I'm eating, at least, the way I'd like to live.

March 22, 1993

Presidential possibilities

Two women, two pins and two compliments from a president. One woman followed her impulse. The other drew back. One feels giddy, the other dumb.

If the president recalls them at all, he remembers neither encounter as vividly as the women do, having relearned two big life lessons: Seize the moment. And to thine own self be true.

On the morning of Bill Clinton's visit to Detroit, both women dressed very deliberately.

Jody Kohn, a manager at Borders Books and Music in Dearborn, knew Clinton would visit the Rouge plant nearby and had a weird premonition she would see him. She put on a skirt and a new green sweater, to which she attached a black velvet pin embroidered in gold and red.

Across town, a Detroit Free Press editor named Renee Murawski, knowing the president would visit her building that day, put on a bright red dress. Being only 5 feet tall, she hoped to stand out from the crowd and win a handshake. She adorned the dress with a pin a friend bought in Moscow — black lacquer with an intricate red design.

Midafternoon at the Free Press, Clinton worked the gaggle of journalists. As he shook Renee's hand, he nodded toward her dress and said, "Nice pin." She flushed with pleasure.

While Clinton met with top editors, Renee sat at her desk replaying his words: Nice pin. Her female friends urged her to give it to him for Hillary, telling her it was the Clintons' 19th anniversary.

But a male friend scoffed: "Don't be silly. It will end up in a box in the basement at the Smithsonian."

She hesitated, clenching the pin in her palm. Then the president stepped onto the elevator and left.

Soon after, stopping at Borders, he chatted with Jody Kohn and admired her pin. "Beautiful," he called it. "Unusual." Where did she buy it?

"I just instinctively took it off and gave it to him," Jody told me. "I said, 'It's your anniversary and you've admired my pin and I'd be thrilled if you gave it to Hillary.' He held it in his hand, studying it, and then he said, 'Well, OK,' and put it in his pocket."

The next morning, when Renee read about Jody, a tidal wave of regret and embarrassment washed over her. "Anybody passes my desk and says, 'Nice banana' and I give it to them," Renee said. "But the president of the United States says 'Nice pin' — and I'm too stupid to hand it over."

Jody, meanwhile, did interviews, took calls from admirers and shrugged off arguments that the president cared no more about her pin than about the lint in his pockets. "He's my president. He can do whatever he wants with my pin."

The rest of us fall into two camps: Sentimentalists believe the president was pin-shopping and did, indeed, give Jody's pin to Hillary. Cynics — including me — believe "Nice pin" is standard presidential small talk.

Renee remains inconsolable. Another woman seized the moment that might have been hers. Jody lost her pin, but gained 15 minutes of fame, an anecdote of presidential proportion, and reason to scrutinize every picture of Hillary's bosom.

Renee, though, gained a ready reply to anyone who ever admires her black lacquer pin from Moscow: "Yes, President Clinton liked it, too. But I wouldn't give it to him, either."

October 16, 1994

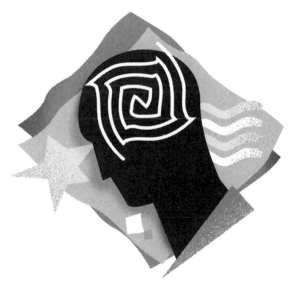

AMBIGUITIES

Searching for the right road

The morning was hazy, and so was I. I had forgotten my wake-up mug of coffee again, but I knew I could trust my autopilot to carry me to the office.

My mind was occupied as usual, with matters more important than the road ahead of me. I listed all the things I hadn't done the day before, all the things I had to do today, all the things I might never do in my lifetime if I didn't get busy.

Suddenly, a swatch of color caught my eye. Just to the left of the highway stood a barn, big and bright red.

"My God!" I thought. "I've driven this route a thousand times and never seen that barn!"

Then, a bit of reason: "Nah," I said. "They must have built it over the weekend."

Within a millisecond, though, the full power of my sluggish morning intellect asserted itself: "There is no way anybody can erect and paint a barn in a weekend."

That left me with only one option. "I am lost."

Whatever I had been musing about vanished, instantly. Only one thing mattered, and mattered completely: To figure out where I was, and find my way back to the right road.

I scanned the horizon. Nothing looked familiar.

Within a heart-pounding minute or two, I spotted an exit sign for a town I knew, and realized I was almost to Brighton. Fifteen minutes earlier, lost in myself, I had taken the wrong fork in the freeway.

I turned around, retraced my path and drove the rest of the way to Detroit with both hands on the steering wheel, hardly blinking. I nodded at each familiar exit like an old woman trying to remind herself she's still with it.

The episode scared me until I began talking with others. They said yes, they, too, get lost on familiar routes regularly. Their eyes are wide open as they drive, but their brains are shut down.

One friend missed his freeway exit on the way home three times in two weeks. Once, he drove half an hour beyond his turnoff before coming to on a strange stretch of highway. Another friend, one evening after work, found himself so lost and confused he had to stop at a gas station to ask directions.

What does it mean when our autopilots shut down? When we can't trust ourselves to get ourselves home? When our horses no longer know the way?

And, when the horse fails — once, twice, three times — shouldn't it be shot?

Perhaps this is an effect of age, except we're not that old. Maybe all those brain cells we murdered years ago with too much alcohol and drugs are finally clogging the circuits.

Or perhaps we have just too many things to think about these days. Beyond the usuals — love, sex, death, money, health, time, food — we've got the stickiest one of all: What do our lives mean anyhow? We're overloaded with questions we can never answer, but which bully their way to the front of our consciousness, short-circuiting our autopilots, confusing our horses.

It all reminds me of something a photographer friend told me months ago: "I think more people are confused than admit it. I'm sure more people are confused than know it. I'm more confused than I should admit. And I act more confused than I really am."

Not me. I'm exactly as lost and confused as I seem.

February 26, 1993

The wrong end of a gun

I went to Gary's Guns last week because I wondered how it felt to sell a gun that one man used to kill another.

I expected to meet people whose business turned my stomach, and whose attitude was tough and cavalier.

Instead, I met two likable people troubled that a shotgun they sold to John Schmitz was used, minutes later, to kill Scott Amedure.

Owners Gary and Nancy Morgan are talking about quitting the business, for reasons beyond Amedure's death. "I'm burned out," Gary says. "I've had it." I didn't expect that. On my way north to the small town of Oxford, I thought about the killing and its curious twists. Everybody still blames the "Jenny Jones" show for provoking Schmitz to kill Amedure, a gay man who confessed his crush on Schmitz during a taping. But why does no one blame those who sold the gun, or manufactured it?

If Jenny Jones gave Schmitz a motive, didn't Gary's Guns give him the means?

For $249.99 plus tax, the Morgans sold him a shotgun and made $45 profit.

As I drove, I imagined hounding gun shops and manufacturers the way zealots hound abortion clinics: Picket them, surround them, harass them, taunt their customers. Drive them out of business.

I was surprised to find Gary's tucked next to a Radio Shack in a bright new strip mall, anchored by Glen's Foods and Blockbuster Video and Arbor Drugs, icons of American enterprise.

I stepped inside a clean, silent, well-lit place, no one smoking, no one cursing, one wall lined with Indian prints and silver jewelry. Then I listened for an afternoon to two people who, no less than any of us, are challenged and confused by guns in America.

"I always thought if we had trouble, it would be for selling a handgun to somebody who used it in a robbery," Gary Morgan told me from behind his counter. "I never thought someone would buy a shotgun and go out and kill someone with it."

Nancy was alone in the store the morning of March 9 when John Schmitz came in, pointed at and bought a shotgun to take hunting, he said, with his dad.

At noon, her brother called about a murder he heard described on his police scanner: a straight guy shot a gay guy who embarrassed him on a talk show.

He asked Nancy, "Were those Carrie's friends?"

Carrie is the Morgans' daughter, and this is the amazing coincidence:

Three weeks before, Carrie, 18, had set up for the "Maury Povich" show an encounter almost identical to the Schmitz-Amedure scene. Carrie and a gay friend confessed their crushes on a straight male acquaintance.

Nancy and Gary Morgan watched and taped the show. "It was kind of cute," Nancy told me. "The guy said, 'I'm straight and I'm happy.' "

She couldn't believe such a funny moment would have sparked violence. Hours later, she learned it was a different talk show, a different pair of men — but the shotgun she had sold that morning.

The phone calls started, cameras came, and everybody asked questions.

I could see the leftover tension in the tightness of her face. I pressed her, wondering if she didn't feel somehow responsible.

"I felt real bad at first," she told me, "but I knew we did nothing wrong."

Still, that first night, Nancy bought a rare six-pack of Bud Light and, sitting alone in the dark at a picnic table in her yard, drank down most of it.

The Morgans are everyday American entrepreneurs who sell guns because they know more about them than about groceries or exercise gizmos.

Gary grew up with guns, on a small Ortonville farm whose men hunted and butchered animals the women cooked and served for dinner.

He and Nancy, married 22 years now, sold hunting guns at

weekend shows for years, considering it a hobby, never owning
more than a few.

They're not the crusty defenders of the gun trade I expected.
They were even naive at first, hoping to carry only long guns —
rifles and shotguns for hunters and target shooters.

But people asked for handguns, so now they carry dozens,
which sell faster than anything else. They sell semiautomatic assault
weapons, too, Uzis and Tec9s, although Nancy feels uneasy about
them: "You can imagine people hiding them under their coats."
Still, she tells me, "People say they enjoy firing them off in their
backyards," then rolls her eyes.

Guns meant pleasure and profit for the Morgans. They had
never been mugged. Or held up. No loved one ever died by a
bullet. As far as they knew, long guns were for hunting, handguns
are tucked under pillows or into purses, and assault weapons —
well, who can say?

They had no problems, no qualms, no real trepidations.

Until now.

The Morgans still wonder why the details of the murder differ in
stories they've read. Not one has had the correct price of the gun,
although they showed every reporter the tag. News people like me
pestered them, and took sly photos from the parking lot, without
even asking.

I tried to explain the challenges of my profession. I didn't want
them to think of us — or me — as malicious. But it takes a lot of talk
— for me, an afternoon in a gun shop — to get beyond the obvious,
beyond our naive expectations of each other.

Take what happened to Nancy four days after the Amedure
killing, while she was bowling in Clawson. A teammate asked: "Did
you sell that gun that killed my stepbrother?"

Nancy couldn't believe it. Never did she imagine selling a gun
that would kill a relative of a friend. After they talked, though,
Nancy felt relieved. The woman didn't seem angry, and said she
wasn't that close to Scott Amedure.

But Nancy had to ask: "Do you still like me?"

From her teammate came the answer she wanted, the one that if
she's human she must want from us all.

She and Gary were putting it behind them. Then, last week, they
learned the 16-year-old boy who took their youngest daughter to

last fall's prom killed himself with his father's shotgun. His mother found him dead in their basement. The medical examiner believes he shot himself in the head deliberately.

The Morgans had not sold that gun. But they grieved for the boy and their daughter, who avoided his funeral.

Finally, last week, Nancy testified at John Schmitz's preliminary examination. She knew they had done nothing unlawful, but still … Her husband reminded her, as he reminded me, that Schmitz could have bought a shotgun from the Kmart down the road.

But he bought it from her.

Nancy had never testified in court. She trembled and paced and felt sick to her stomach.

She will probably have to testify at the trial. And maybe again if, as they fear, Amcdure's survivors sue them.

Gary sighs. "You know what Schmitz should've done? He should have taken that money and gone down to Pontiac or Detroit and got a couple goons to come and just rough that guy up.

"He didn't have to do what he did."

As I'm asking questions, a regular customer who overhears begins to rant about the liberal press, then Nazis, and Bill Clinton, and taking away people's guns until they're just numbers, slaves of the state, vulnerable to anyone. The liberal press, he says, exaggerates the menace of guns.

"Somebody could run over 80 people with a car, but you can't shoot more than six people with a revolver without reloading it!" he shouts at me.

Nancy seems embarrassed. I'm relieved when he's gone, after buying a rifle scope. He's the kind of gun nut any of us might fear.

The Morgans are not like him. But neither, in this business, can they afford to be afraid of him, or to turn him away.

"If I had it to do over again," Gary says of his shop, "I wouldn't. I'd go into business again, but not guns. There's too many headaches dealing with the public. People come in with bad attitudes, and they hassle you. People come in and order guns and then change their minds. They figure you're rich."

He's curious, too, why in all his years of knowing gun dealers, he has never heard a single one talk about having sold a gun that killed someone. "Even my brother," he says, as if thinking aloud.

"He owns a shop in the UP. I wonder if he's ever sold a gun that was used in a crime."

Preparing to leave, I can no longer imagine picketing the Morgans. Until Congress changes its mind, they have a right to make money from guns. The rest of us can only hope that the guns they sell will kill nothing more noble than a deer.

Or that they quit the business, and find equal profits in some other commodity of American life.

I'm about to go when the phone rings.

Gary answers, listens and seems flustered. He pulls from a file a yellow form, the one all gun-buyers must sign, attesting that they are not felons or fugitives or drug addicts.

"Can I ask why this gun is in question?" Gary asks stiffly.

Then, "Nobody was shot with it, were they?"

When he hangs up he buries his face in his hands. "Doggone it."

A handgun he sold was used in a crime. The caller, from the Bureau of Alcohol, Tobacco and Firearms, couldn't or wouldn't say what crime or how much pain and grief rippled from it.

Gary lowers his hands and looks straight at me, and his eyes look moist as he says:

"Now I'm going to be wondering what this gun did. Later tonight, it'll be on my mind."

Nancy, beside him behind the counter, sighs.

April 9, 1995

Snap judgment, suspect verdict

I tell this story in slow motion because that is the only way to show you how fickle my judgments were, how swiftly I ricocheted between stereotypes and modern sensibilities.

I have replayed this moment many times. I wanted to do right — to think right — but did not know how. Judge for yourself.

I am visiting one of my favorite small women's shops in the town where I live, a town mostly white, but with a solid minority of Asian-, Hispanic- and African-Americans.

The owner and I are reminiscing about San Francisco, where both of us once lived. We are about the same age. We wear the same kind of loose unstructured clothing, the sort the shop sells. Just functional, natural fabrics to cover your body.

Suddenly, in the middle of a sentence, the owner turns toward the only other customers in the shop, a couple I had not noticed: a very heavy black woman, sloppily dressed in polyester, and her companion, a tall, emaciated black man with hollow cheeks and a pronounced stoop.

I think: He must be a heroin addict. I think: They don't belong here. I think: I've never seen anyone who looks like them in this store.

Then I think: Shame on you. Maybe he has AIDS. Maybe they're new in town and don't know that this store carries no clothes like the clothes they're wearing.

By this time, the proprietor has taken 10 steps toward them. The black woman looks her in the eye and says, loudly: "You think I'm here to steal."

I think: Uh-oh. This could get ugly. The proprietor says: "No, I don't think you're here to steal, but I saw you walk in with an empty paper bag, and now I see it has something in it. May I look?"

I silently beg the proprietor to back away, to stop before she humiliates the two black customers, and herself, too.

The woman says: "No, you can't see inside! I have my rights."

I think: Whoa, she's ballsy. Then I think: Well, she does have her rights. She's being accused of shoplifting, and she has every right in the world to stand up to this arrogant white shopkeeper, who moments earlier I had liked so much.

The proprietor persists: "Is there something private inside that you don't want me to see?"

The black woman replies: "Yes!'

I think: Isn't she pushing this too far? Why not open the bag and vindicate herself?

Before my judgments can ricochet again, the skinny man and the fat woman turn and run. Straight out the door. Wobbly and unsteady, they run out the door and down the street, and I think, full of sadness: Guilty as charged.

Later a friend wonders whether the black couple were just fed up with having been eyed too often in their lives, and ran to get away from suspicion and trouble.

I hadn't even thought of that.

But later, when I returned to the shop, the owner told me she found two leather eyeglass cases missing, each worth $35. The police had picked up the skinny guy, wanted on another charge, but never found the woman. Or the merchandise.

The owner told me she, too, had felt conflicted that day, just as I had, her mind hopscotching over all sorts of fears and uncertainties.

"You have to rely on your instincts now," she told me, "because your intellect is so muddled."

Bewildered by this episode, I, too, wished I might have made an easy judgment that held, that made me feel sure and secure. But it also seems none of us should feel shame for second-guessing ourselves, for being not quite sure, for being wary of any assumption that cannot, for the sake of a human being, be budged.

April 4, 1995

Accidental, but everlasting

Imagine you are a 14-year-old girl, spirited and venturesome, and responsible for the death of a friend who fell off the hood of a car while you, in play, were driving.

Imagine you are a father carrying a plate of just-grilled burgers into the house when you stumble and plunge the fork in your hand through the heart of your little son.

Imagine you are a hunter, careful in every respect, except for the morning you pull the trigger in groggy haste and end the life of your best friend.

We read about the 14-year-old in our newspapers. Over the years we have read about the others, and more, including the driver who couldn't dodge a 10-year-old girl dashing to school and killed her.

Imagine having to live with yourself after such a tragedy: responsible for the hole in someone else's life, while ministering to a hole in your own.

We do not recognize them, but people who have accidentally killed other people live and work among us, carrying a secret load of grief and guilt. I personally know two. One's car struck a boy on a bicycle. Another's car slid on black ice on a rural Michigan highway and plowed into the only other car on the road, killing an 80-year-old woman.

They cannot recognize each other, either, which is too bad, because there are no support groups for them. Each year, they get through the anniversaries of the accidents alone while, somewhere else, the family and friends of the ones who died mourn and wonder. Despite an intellectual understanding that "accidents happen," they cannot help but lay tentative blame: "She should have ... Why didn't he ...? If only ..."

That someone you love dies because of a fluke, a flicker, a trip, a slip, a momentary glance in the wrong direction is impossible. Does it take so little to end so precious a life? Shouldn't a 10-page report be offered, a complex and reasonable explanation?

Not, "Her foot slipped, and that was that." Or, "He could not stop in time."

One of my clearest memories is my own near-membership in this secret society of accidental killers.

On a gray November afternoon, I was idling at a stop sign, waiting to pull onto a busy road. I glanced right. I glanced left. The way was clear.

I pressed the accelerator and oh my God a boy on a bicycle and I slammed on the brake and he tumbled from the bike and my heart stopped my breath stopped my life stopped.

I could not unglue myself from my seat. A thousand questions filled my head: Why didn't you look twice? What will you say to his mother? What will you say to your mother? How can you compensate his family? How can they go on? How can you go on?

I found the boy sitting on the concrete in front of my car, stunned but unhurt. Neither of us could be sure our vehicles had collided, but he had swerved violently when my car began to move. He assumed I had seen him.

I apologized. I wrote my name and number on a slip of paper for him to give his mother. I hugged him and teased him and tried to make light of it. He pedaled away, unruffled.

But all the way home I sobbed, for the difference a split second would have made, for the sorry explanation I would have had to make, the boy's family would have had to hear, and we all would have had to live with: "It just happened."

October 6, 1994

Conditional surrender to sex

We were alone beneath the stars, high in the mountains, miles from the nearest light, our sleeping bags unrolled on the ground, weary from a long drive and anticipating sleep.

Or so I thought.

We were not lovers, merely acquaintances. We worked together. We respected each other. He owned a few acres in the mountains, and I admired that back-to-the-land streak in anyone. So we agreed to make this weekend camping trip together to his patch of earth.

A few days earlier, oh so briefly, I thought about saying something. Issuing a "don't-get-any-ideas" warning. But I didn't. I thought he'd feel insulted.

He did not worry so much about my feelings.

For hours on that starlit night he pestered me. Stroked me. Whispered to me first, then argued, then whined: "Oh, come on. You'll love it. Why'd you come up here with me then? Just once. It's such a beautiful night. You'll enjoy it, really. Come on. Please?"

I didn't scream, because there was no one to hear. I didn't fight, because there was nowhere to run. It was his car, and he had the keys. Instead, I curled up. I buried my head against my chest while he touched me. I slapped blindly at his touches, as if I were batting away mosquitoes.

Because this happened more than a decade ago, I can't remember with precision how long he continued. I wore no watch that night.

All I know is that he went on forever. Unrelenting.

Finally, weary and weepy, I gave up. I remember the sting of my tears rolling down my cheeks and into my ears as I lay on my back and he moaned.

Then, I fell instantly into sleep, as if from the top of a mountain.

Our weekend ended early, because I was sullen and that made

him angry. There was nothing to say on the long ride home.

I never called what happened that night "rape." I still don't.

But it wasn't bliss, either.

I wonder why it has no name. Because it happens all the time: Men push. Women submit.

No violence, no shouting. Just sadness and defeat.

How many of us women have watched this sort of thing happen to us, as if we were outside our bodies, in the 30 years since a confluence of factors made sexual interaction easier, at least practically speaking?

That night in the mountains I surrendered for one reason: I was tired and wanted to escape.

But we surrender for reasons besides fatigue.

■ Duty: Some women may feel an obligation to reward men who've been particularly kind, or patient, or ardent. Other women may feel an obligation to be a good-and-ready wife.

■ Ambiguity: Part of us wants sex, the other part is wary. And as the train is moving toward the station, so to speak, we're still not sure. We may surrender at the same moment that we conclude, "No, this is stupid."

Some men claim not to understand this. But most women know there is a vast geography of shifting sentiment between Yes and No.

■ Hope: Sometimes we surrender because our disinterest might turn into delight. A friend calls this the "No-but-I-could-be-convinced" approach. Sometimes it works. Often it doesn't, and we wonder why we gave in.

We make these excuses for our surrenders, but that's no consolation for the vanquished.

Years after that night in the mountains, I'm surprised to find how angry I am about it. Angrier than I was then. At both him and me, and the games people play.

Now, wiser and less polite, I would not whimper but shout. Not for help, but for my own integrity — to let him know how I felt about his boorish presumptions.

I would surrender only if he held me down and forced me. Then I could call it rape.

March 22, 1992

Reality: true or false?

By the time O.J. Simpson finished his TV interview the other night, I had a headache from squinting at him, trying to spot falsehood on his face as he spoke with a credible self-confidence.

All I wanted to do was go to bed and suspend my exhausting search for Truth.

The night before, listening to Bill Clinton on TV, I felt some optimism about the state of the union. But when a friend criticized the speech as "intellectually dishonest," I thought: The president lied? I believed words he didn't believe himself?

When I challenged my friend for evidence of dishonesty, he threw a few facts at me about Clinton's record. I threw a few facts back. Neither of us had any idea whose facts were better or if any of our facts were true.

We acknowledged that neither of us knew all the facts about Clinton. Or anything else. If we knew all the facts, could we know the Truth?

I put my head in my hands.

I'm so tired of looking for Truth. I feel foolish for believing it exists, buried somewhere like a shiny penny in a pile of dead leaves.

Here's the problem: I grew up thinking that most people were honest and that lying was a sin. You could tell a liar by shifty eyes and beads of sweat and a voice that stammered and cracked. Easy.

Later, as a reporter, I plodded through records and interviews, learning that Truth emerges from complex situations in flakes, not chunks.

Now, as a news consumer, I am inundated with facts I did not collect. I am nudged this way and that by spin doctors and opinion columnists. I am called, with the nation, to decide:

■ Anita Hill or Clarence Thomas?

■ William Kennedy Smith or Patty Bowman?
■ O.J. Simpson or Marcia Clark?
■ Bill Clinton or his challengers?
■ Hillary or her critics?
Rarely are these national dilemmas resolved in a satisfying way.

Richard Nixon's tapes did him in, and Susan Smith confessed, but most liars don't. And lately it seems people lie more nimbly than before. They go on TV to explain themselves and sound honest as fresh snow.

I envy my friends who can decide without anguish whom to distrust. "I've got all the facts I need," they say. I never have all the facts I need. I flail in a sea of facts with no inner tube of Truth.

What frightens me most is the possibility that although no one is telling the Truth, no one is lying either. They say what they think is true, while impartial observers recognize it as false.

But can a man rape or kill a woman, then deny it — without losing his mind or sprouting a huge pimple on his nose?

Yes. Liars come before the nation all the time with clear complexions and well-crafted speeches, indistinguishable from bearers of Truth.

Wise people, I suspect, abandon the Truth-seeking game. Why chew on the details of the life of someone who will never have dinner at your house?

As I age, I realize how little I know for sure, but I'd like to feel less troubled by that. Better to spend energy examining the lies I tell myself and counting the few scraps of Truth I can own:

My hands are cold. My coffee is hot. The ring on my finger is round.

January 28, 1996

Peacemaker in black and white

The house sits on a quiet, well-tended corner in Bloomfield Township, on a street named Wilshire with sloping lawns and no sidewalks. It has a family room, a master bath, neutral decorating and a two-way fireplace.

When Birmingham real estate agent Carole Pray listed it for $179,000 last November, she knew from 18 years' experience that it would sell quickly.

Indeed, by dusk on the very first day, a full-price offer had come in — but it was rejected.

Within 24 hours, trouble began.

Pray, a white woman, was accused of racial discrimination. Despite phone calls and pleas to work things out, she could not fix what seemed a terrible misunderstanding.

Within weeks, the conflict grew. Soon, she was charged in U.S. District Court with violating federal fair housing laws. A retired black couple from Southfield, Eddie and Jacquelyn Jackson, demanded $1 million in damages.

All the newspapers wrote it up.

Stunned, she found herself the center of attention — a woman who for years had taught other agents about fair housing laws and started a program in Pontiac to help low-income people find good housing deals.

Her friends sent her sympathetic notes: "There but for the grace of God go all of us." "Carole Pray a racist? Absurd!" A swirl of emotions and dry legal actions sucked her into what she came to call "a river of sadness."

Then one night Pray heard on her home answering machine the voice of a man who identified himself as "Jim Sumpter, federal investigator." In despair she thought, "What more can happen to me?"

But it was Sumpter who saved her — and the Jacksons, too —

from a long, anguishing federal court fight. In a week, he achieved what high-priced attorneys and judges and a plodding court system might have chewed on for months.

Sumpter is an unlikely hero, a black man with a gold badge who in a thicket of racial accusations, denials and hurt feelings was able to find a path to peace.

In the end, nobody lost. Nobody won, either, exactly what they wanted.

But they won enough to stop squabbling.

Sumpter's secret? He listened.

"Let me formally introduce myself," he says as he slides into the booth of a restaurant where we agreed to meet. He flips open a leather case to flash badge and says, "Jim Sumpter. Federal investigator."

He grew up in Detroit, but works out of Chicago, one of 12 investigators for the Fair Housing Enforcement Division of the U.S. Department of Housing and Urban Development.

He is a big man with a moustache who dresses in black. He drives a 10-year-old black Cadillac across the Midwest, its backseat piled with old magazines and law journals and enough fresh clothes for a few days.

He earns $52,000 a year investigating the behaviors that discourage people from buying, moving into or living peacefully in the homes of their choice. He specializes in the ugliest of those behaviors: Cross-burnings. Firebombings. Verbal threats by angry neighbors. Police inaction.

All illegal.

He interviews racist thugs and gang members and white supremacists and cops. He wears shades and sits with his arms crossed over his chest and looks people in the eye.

This promotes truth-telling, he says.

This leads even bad guys, he says, to brag about their badness and, eventually, to reveal whatever fear or ignorance compelled it.

That gives Jim Sumpter something to work with. Because he prefers, if he can and if the situation allows, to resolve problems rather than collect evidence to prosecute them. His bosses prefer that, too, because it's quicker and cheaper for the taxpayer.

Sumpter considers himself good at conciliation, and guess what adjective he says best describes him? Not "intimidating." Not "tough." Not "mean."

"Sensitive."

Indeed, on his official government business card, under his name and next to his official title of "Investigator," he has added his own self-description: "Negotiator."

The Jacksons' lawsuit and a complaint they filed with HUD landed on Sumpter's desk. Here's what they say happened:

Arriving early to take a look at the Wilshire house, they parked at the curb to wait for their real estate agent.

As they sat in their car, they watched a white woman pull up, walk into the house, then, a few minutes later, leave the house and drive away.

She looked them right in the eye.

When they toured the home a few minutes later, they loved it and that evening made a full-price offer.

The suit says their offer was never presented to the home's owner. The woman who looked them in the eye was Carole Pray, they contend. She wrote "REFUSED" in big letters across their offer, in her distinctively beautiful handwriting, and jotted her client's initials beneath it.

She treated them this way because they are black, and tried to buy into a mostly white neighborhood.

"I am still having nightmares and recurring dreams over the ordeal," Mrs. Jackson, who is retired from the Ford Motor Credit Corp., told a reporter. "I was simply trying to fulfill a dream of purchasing a nice home in a nice neighborhood."

Her husband, a retired maintenance superintendent at Wayne State University, added: "I guess some people still feel they can treat blacks like second-class citizens."

Jim Sumpter's 55 years have taught him wisdom and savvy.

Among the things he knows: Discrimination is hateful and painful and wrong. But not everything that looks like discrimination is.

He grew up on Detroit's east side, graduating from high school without being able to read. He taught himself with books he bought at Goodwill.

As a young man he worked with gang members on Detroit's

southwest side, trying to talk them out of violence and self-destruction. His office was in a former funeral home; his first desk was an embalming table.

He liked to wave his arm at the leftover caskets and say to young thugs, "Hey man, you don't have far to go!"

When he was 23, he says, he went to work for Wonder Bread as its first black delivery truck driver, against the wishes of the drivers' union.

"For a year I drove that big white bread truck empty, so whites and blacks could see me and get used to a black man behind the wheel," he says. "I took the abuse, the curses, the name-calling from the union, too."

When he finally began delivering bread, white suburban store owners "spit on me, knocked the bread out of my hands."

"But you begin to not take it so personally. You're on a mission. I was making it better for the young people who now drive a bread truck, whose positions were paid for by those kinds of dues."

Later he worked for the City of Ann Arbor as its sole investigator of housing discrimination and police brutality, long before laws banned it. There, he earned most of a bachelor's degree from the University of Michigan and gained investigative skills he has used, for 20 years now, for various arms of the federal government.

Much of what he learned about "the system," though, he learned at the elbow of George Romney, whom he met in 1962 when Romney was running for Michigan governor. "He took me under his wing," Sumpter says, and he traveled with Romney, worked security for him, even accompanied him to the Republican National Convention in 1968.

Once, as Romney and Sumpter stood just outside a Detroit auditorium, an elderly woman approached Romney, in his dark blue suit and well-coiffed hair, and, mistaking him for a building employee, handed him a letter to mail.

Then secretary of the United States Department of Housing and Urban Development, Romney shrugged, walked the letter over to a mailbox and dropped it in.

Sumpter will tell that story to you over and over again if you want to hear it. It left a very deep mark on him because he, too, has been mistaken for someone he isn't.

"Sometimes," he says, "going into restaurants, or standing outside a club, people will walk up and hand me the keys to their cars.

"I could become very indignant. But I remember that lesson.

"Others' perception of you, or the situation you're standing in — you can't become adversely impacted by it. If you do, you become empoisoned."

When Jim Sumpter arrived in Detroit to investigate the Jacksons' complaint, he knew everyone involved would feel overwhelmed, intimidated and helpless.

"These things just take on a life of their own," he says. "They grow, like malignancies."

So he tried to move quickly.

The Jacksons at first would not meet with him, but Carole Pray told him everything, crying into a wad of tissues she kept in her purse.

It was not she who saw the Jacksons at the curb that day.

In fact, she didn't even know they were black until she read newspaper accounts of their lawsuit.

They're wrong to say she didn't present their offer. She called her client and talked to him about it. She encouraged him to reject it because the Jacksons had put down only $1,000 in earnest money — in that area, $7,000 or more would be more typical, she said. "Our philosophy is: Weak deposit, weak offer."

Yes, she admitted, she had written "REFUSED" on the offer, and added her client's initials, but only with his consent.

Then she told the Jacksons' agent simple ways the deal could be saved — making, in effect, a counteroffer.

Whether that agent ever relayed that message to the Jacksons, she didn't know. She never heard back from any of them — except when they accused her of discrimination.

She and the Jacksons had never met or spoken.

Sumpter listened and watched her and asked a few questions.

Then he said: "I can tell by your face that you believe what you tell me.

"And if what you say is true, you may be a victim, too."

That night in his motel room, Sumpter, a man too big to work from a double bed, got down on the floor, spreading around him every sworn statement collected by every lawyer in the case. Then he read every word.

Included was a statement from another real estate agent who said it was she who stopped by the Wilshire house and saw the Jacksons in their car.

No matter who the Jacksons had seen, Sumpter knew enough to know no discrimination had occurred.

Carole Pray had sworn under oath she presented their offer. Her client swore he heard and rejected it, but made a counteroffer. Even the Jacksons' agent agreed.

What had happened? Was it an innocent mistake? A misunderstanding? Miscommunication? Something else entirely?

Jim Sumpter didn't know and didn't care. It just seemed ridiculous to him it had dragged out this long — six months already.

"What was unusual about this case," Sumpter told me, "was that it was so simple. It was all right there! Why didn't the attorneys do something? Why were these families allowed to hurt for so long?

"They were in the same situation. They were all good people suffering."

Within a week, it was over.

Sumpter demanded a meeting with the Jacksons. He drove to their new home, the one they bought after the Wilshire deal didn't work out. Because their carpet was fresh and new, he took off his shoes at the door, sat down on their living room floor and spread on their coffee table all the sworn statements.

He told them his conclusion: Yes, they felt discriminated against. No, they were not wrong to sue or complain. But it did not appear they had been discriminated against, either.

They conceded he was right.

We just want out, they told him.

But they were afraid that Carole Pray and her realty company, Max Broock Inc., might countersue and really trap them.

So he went back to Carole Pray and asked her what she wanted.

"My spirit is broken," she told him. She didn't even feel anger, just numbness and pain. She, too, wanted it to be over.

But she also wanted her good name back.

No man can return to anyone a lost reputation, or lost dignity. But Sumpter did his best.

Acting as negotiator and intermediary, Sumpter helped these black and white people, who never spoke or met, compose a five-page document all three could sign.

It said the Jacksons filed suit only because they felt their rights had been violated. They "regret any embarrassment, humiliation, harm or damage" their lawsuit caused Carole Pray, and "now understand that her behavior was ethical and professional."

All suits and complaints would be dismissed. And everyone promised not to sue each other anymore.

"You mean it's over?" Mr. Jackson asked Jim Sumpter after he signed his name.

"It's over," Sumpter told him.

"Now I can rest," Mr. Jackson sighed. "Now I can sleep at night."

Jim Sumpter left the Jacksons' home that evening tired and hungry, and slipped into a Boston Market just before it closed, in time for a chicken pot pie to celebrate another day's work done.

In the months since, Carole Pray has published a book of religious poems inspired mostly by restless nights.

At 52, she is retired from real estate, not sure what she'll do next. But she credits Jim Sumpter with giving her the chance to even think about a future. She sent him her book, and wants him to come by for dinner the next time he's around.

He has promised he would.

The Jacksons, who did not want to be interviewed, live in a condo in Farmington Hills. They, too, have invited Sumpter to dinner and, much to his surprise, sent a note of praise to his boss that mentioned his "kindness and consideration" and his hard work.

"We just want to say thank you for assigning our case to Mr. Sumpter," their letter said, "and may God continue to bless each and every one."

As for the nice house on Wilshire:

It eventually sold for about $15,000 less than its asking price to a company that buys homes of transferred workers.

Who lives there now?

No one knows, and no one cares.

October 22, 1995

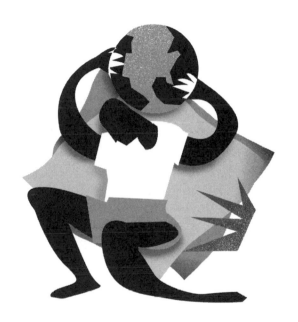

LOSING & WINNING

Hoop schemes

A friend and I once entertained ourselves at a boring minor-league baseball game by trying to decide which pro sport is the best metaphor for real life.

"Football," I remember saying. "Nasty and brutish."

"Baseball," he said. "Mostly nothing happens. You have opportunities to do something significant, but usually you don't."

Finally we settled on basketball: Running and sweating. Lots of flukes. Many ways to score, but people always grabbing at you, trying to disrupt your dribble, eager to ruin your chances.

I thought about the flukiness of basketball and life after I heard about two guys who live miles apart and never met, but flirted with the same fate on separate basketball courts.

One worked hard to seduce fate. The other winged it.

First, Bobby Shivar.

His wife entered him in a contest at a Kmart near their home in Beulaville, N.C. Sponsored by Gillette, the contest offered one American one chance to shoot a basket from the 3-point line at the NCAA Final Four championship — and win a million bucks.

Bobby is 45, a pipe fitter, earning $32,000 a year. When he heard last August that the chance was his, that he beat out two million contenders, he began, as any man would, to practice.

He planted a hoop on his gravel driveway, stood there and shot — sometimes missing 10 out of 10. Gillette kindly sent former Boston Celtics star Dave Cowens to coach Bobby, helping him work his success rate up to 40 percent.

The big day came — coincidentally his wife's 42nd birthday. Bobby raised his arms to the cheering crowd at New Orleans' Lakefront Arena, bounced the basketball three times and shot.

It clanked off the rim. The crowd groaned.

And Bobby went home, to his old job, his old car, his old life, his getting-older wife.

End of story.

Meanwhile, in a Chicago suburb, a guy with a ticket to that night's Chicago Bulls-Miami Heat game realized he couldn't go. He handed the ticket to his friend, a 23-year-old office supply salesman named Don Calhoun.

Don wasn't a Bulls regular — he'd been to one game in six years. But as he strolled into Chicago Stadium, two young women on the lookout for a random fan noticed his mustard-yellow suede shoes, size 13, which he'd bought for $54.99 from Kinney.

They told him they loved his shoes. And you, they said, will win a million dollars if you can sink a basket from the opposite foul line — 76 feet down the court.

"I was skeptical at first," Don said. "I thought I had to pay some money or something."

But no. This was a year-long promotion by Coca-Cola and a local restaurant chain. All Don had to do was stand there at half-time, thousands of eyes upon him, and throw the ball.

Hard.

Don plays basketball with a YMCA league, but he does more passing than shooting. He figured he'd launch the ball off his chest, but a cheerleader promised him better luck if he threw it like a baseball.

So he did, giving it his best heave.

Across the court it flew, in a high, elegant arc that ended as the ball swished through the net.

Suddenly, Don was rich, his life ignited with new possibilities, his 3-year-old son more likely to succeed. All thanks to a string of flukes: a free ticket, yellow suede shoes, a word from a cheerleader, the sudden strength in his arm.

Bulls star Michael Jordan said this about Don's shot: "God works in mysterious ways."

Maybe that's the moral of these stories: No amount of practice can direct the mysterious moves of God, a basketball or a life.

April 19, 1993

Singular thoughts, all alone

We kiss good-bye on the sidewalk in front of the terminal, the engine idling in the car beside us.

In minutes, a contraption with wings will take him away from me, while I travel in a contraption with wheels. Either trip could hurt or kill one of us, and hours or days could pass before the other would know.

I think of these things as I drive away, a hollowness in my chest. His leave-takings do this to me every time, stirring up forebodings and dark fantasies about life alone.

I grew up in a household that took good-byes seriously. No one ever said it aloud, but the point of good-byes, we all knew, was to express the affection you might not get a chance to express again.

None of us left the house, even for a quick trip to the dime store, without kissing good-bye. Even now, when we grown kids leave my parents' home, the same one we grew up in, my mother and father stand at the picture window in their living room and wave as we pull from the driveway.

We wave back. If it's dark, we flash the headlights.

It's a routine as hallowed as grace before supper.

When my partner and I kiss at the airport, I leave thinking it ought to have lasted longer. It ought to have been deeper. We ought to have said more. Because this could be it, the end of our years together.

Usually I head to work from the airport and forget for a few hours. Until later, when I return to an empty home.

I turn the key and open the door. As always, I am startled that absolutely nothing has changed since that morning.

My slippers are where I left them. The half-filled coffeepot, its contents cold, sits on the sink. The papers lie scattered on the coffee table. No new lights are burning, no CD is playing, nothing simmers on the stove.

The mail is still in the box.

There's only me here, and nothing will move or change or clean itself or mess itself up unless I do it.

I wonder how people who live alone cope. Maybe that's what pets are for: to rumple a rug, crumple a newspaper, leave a little mess. Something new, anything new.

My mood picks up as I consider dinner. A wisp of freedom rises in me. I might choose popcorn and bourbon in bed. Or half a grapefruit. Or I might sprawl on the couch with a bagful of slivered almonds watching CNN for hours on end — an idiosyncrasy he finds maddening.

Tomorrow, I suspect, I'll remember how it is to be single, and take myself out to breakfast with the Free Press and the New York Times. The day ahead will be entirely mine: no one else to consider.

Tonight, I know, I can read a book in bed till 4 a.m., or stay on the phone all night with my friends, or clean out my closet, or bake a middle-of-the-night cheesecake, with no comment from him, no wish — his or mine — that I be with him in bed.

Instead, it grows late, and I tire more quickly than expected and move to bed. But I don't close my eyes.

Years ago I read about a survey that surprised researchers: Many professional women admitted they slept poorly when they traveled out of town, away from their bed partners. Then, I thought that was pretty pathetic. Now, I am one of those women, unable to find easy comfort, even in a familiar bed, when he isn't in it.

So, instead of sleeping, I lie on my back, on his side of the bed, and think about the years ahead of us, ahead of me. I guess this is practice, a rehearsal for a time when I might be alone, in a house that's all mine, only mine, every day without him, only me.

January 22, 1993

Hurrah for the loser

When my TV told me the other morning that Anthony Young had lost another one, I sat up in bed and cheered.

"I love this guy! What an inspiration!"

Some athletes feel sorry for this New York Mets pitcher who just broke an 82-year-old record by pitching 24 straight losing games.

I don't understand the pity. He doesn't seem to feel sorry for himself, which is why he's such a joy to watch. He may pitch again Saturday and, frankly, I'm rooting for another loss.

Some of us might have quit after 10 or 15. We might have developed a nagging flu, or severe muscle aches, or a case of amnesia that prevented us from figuring out how we ended up in Tahiti or how to get home. Young has engineered no such schemes.

He has suited up, game after game, hurled the damn baseball and lost, game after game.

I admire Young because he's disproving that old Vince Lombardi line: "Winning isn't everything. It's the only thing." Look at what losing has won him: He's surrounded by reporters seeking quotes and little kids seeking autographs. He's received hundreds of letters, even good-luck charms. He's the apple of every announcer's eye.

And he's become a star.

Why? Anthony Young, he's us. He's who we are inside, beneath the bluster. He's us in fifth grade, unable to last even one round in the spelling bee. He's us in ninth grade, reliably clumsy on the dance floor. He's us in 10th grade, tongue-tied and pimply and sure no one would ever love us.

And he's the adult we are now: Day after day losing our little battles with age, flab, ineptitude, insignificance. Waking up each morning confident this day will be different, then watching once again as the ball we pitch with all our might gets knocked out of the park.

Our options: To sulk. To curse. To hide. To beat up on ourselves or some other handy target.

Or to shrug it off like Anthony Young.

Asked if he isn't feeling humiliated, Young smiled and said, "It's not embarrassing. Someone has to win, and someone has to lose. I'm just losing." He said he doesn't dwell on it away from the park, adding, as if he's never heard of the secret pleasure of obsessive self-pity: "Why keep thinking about it?"

His manager, Dallas Green, sounds more wise, too, than many of those whose job it is to pat our fannies as we trot into the fray. Said Green of his losing pitcher: "I tell him the sun will keep coming up. It rained early today, but the sun broke through."

The philosopher Nietzsche said, or at least I've spent my adulthood thinking he said, "If it doesn't kill you, it'll make you stronger." Anthony Young's defeats haven't killed or maimed him. And consider what he's learned.

That life goes on, and so does the play-by-play. That losing a few games makes you a goat, but losing a lot turns you into a hero. And that no matter if you win or lose, you can always go home and grill a fine steak in the backyard.

What happy lessons. What a happy story.

July 1, 1993

Let evening come

The day I read that poet Jane Kenyon had died, I did something I have never done: I tried to call her husband, to say I don't know what.

I never met either Kenyon or her partner, poet Donald Hall. But through their spare words I feel I have come to know them.

They lived in an old family farmhouse in a tiny town in New Hampshire. Both wrote about the simple life around them — toads and peonies and wood thrushes — and the more complicated life, too — men and women doing common work in uncommon circumstances.

Poetry has lost its reputation in this country. It's slow. It's sometimes obscure. You must sit still for it.

That's why I'm reading it again.

Today would have been Jane Kenyon's 48th birthday. She was born in Ann Arbor and met Hall there, as his student at the University of Michigan. They left in 1975 for a simpler life.

Her death from leukemia shocked me because he was to be the one who died first. He is 66, and six years ago was diagnosed with liver cancer, which she wrote about, and so did he, especially in his book of essays called "Life Work."

I remember best from "Life Work" Hall's description of a good day, including lunch in bed with his wife — cheese, bread, V-8 and raisins — then a 20-minute nap for each of them, then making love.

Theirs seemed the best possible life: writing, tending the garden, walking the dog, listening to birds. Indolent lunches in bed. But I knew she struggled with serious depression, too, writing after one successful treatment of awakening at dawn: "Easeful air presses through the screen with the wild, complex song of the bird, and I am overcome by ordinary contentment. What hurt me so terribly all my life until this moment?"

The night of the day I read Jane Kenyon's obituary, I picked up the phone, and dialed directory information for their town.

Their phone rang busy. And as I tried another half-dozen times, it rang busy over and over again.

I had no clue what I would say. What does a stranger know about grief? I have lost only the expectation of more words from her, and an image of them together in a house outside whose windows peonies bloom — "staggered," she wrote, "by their own luxuriance."

Instead, I wrote a note addressed to Donald Hall, Eagle Pond, Wilmot Flat, N.H. Sometimes, I said, we have no clue how far our words ripple and what they stir. I told him his wife's work had reached me. I am sorry she is gone.

I imagine notes piling up on his desk, spilling onto the floor, words from strangers affirming Jane Kenyon's life and his own. I hope he can accept them as gifts that require no more words from him.

Here is one of Jane Kenyon's poems, written at dusk.

Let the light of late afternoon
shine through chinks in the barn moving
up the bales as the sun moves down.
Let the cricket take up chafing
as a woman takes up her needles
and her yarn. Let evening come.

Let dew collect on the hoe abandoned
in long grass. Let the stars appear
and the moon disclose her silver horn.

Let the fox go back to its sandy den.
Let the wind die down. Let the shed
go black inside. Let evening come.
To the bottle in the ditch, to the scoop
in the oats, to air in the lung
Let evening come.

Let it come, as it will, and don't
be afraid. God does not leave us
comfortless, so let evening come.

May 23, 1995

World-class flukes

The other morning, when his driveway was slippery with snow, a friend accidentally crashed his car through his garage door, taking down the door and a good chunk of his garage wall.

Not only did he bang up his knee and his head and sprain his back, but all the next day he beat himself up for his stupidity. (The story is complicated, but suffice it to say he made one tiny mistake.)

"Nonsense," I said, being a supportive friend. "It was just a moment of stupidity in a lifetime of reason and sound judgment."

"Right," he said, groaning. "Nobody remembers all the mornings I didn't smash my car into my garage."

"Exactly," I replied. "Look at what happens to these Olympic athletes. They're the very best in their sports, and they break all kinds of records, but then they get to the Olympics and BLAM! A mini-second of distraction, or a speck of something on their visors, and that's the end of their Olympic dream."

I quoted what I heard American luger Duncan Kennedy say after he spun out at 80 m.p.h.: "I crashed at the Olympics. What can you say?"

What can you say except that sport, like life, ain't fair?

There is no Lifetime Achievement in Luge award.

The NCAA championship goes not to the college basketball team with the best free-throw percentage over the season, but to the one whose guy on the line at the last moment of the last game actually gets the ball through the hoop.

A fraction of an inch off and BLAM! No basket, no point, no championship.

Dan Jansen is acknowledged to be the fastest skater in the world, but his skate slips and BLAM, he's out of contention and commentators try to pin down a "mistake."

But it didn't look like a mistake to me. It looked like a fluke.

Like all of us, Olympians want to believe they control their environments. They work hard at it and nothing else, practicing daily, training the body and the mind to perform in a limited arena — a rink, a slope, an icy run.

They become so skilled that the difference between a champion and an also-ran comes down to distinctions the eye can hardly see.

Is it not amazing that the Norwegian favored to win the gold in downhill skiing lost to Tommy Moe by four one-hundredths of a second?

How long is that? It is the length of time a car traveling 60 m.p.h. needs to cover 3½ feet.

It is briefer than the blink of an eye, which ophthalmologists say requires 25 one-hundredths of a second.

Centuries ago, the Greeks could not measure it. Now we can and do. Imagine how tiny is the fluke that costs a skier four one-hundredths of a second.

They say the Olympic Games celebrate achievement, but from what I can tell, they celebrate the inevitability of flukes.

Even Olympic athletes, having mastered every micro-factor of themselves and their environments, encounter a bump, a speck, a twitch, a blink that throws them off, spins them out and humbles them.

So my friend, who has hardly mastered his own driveway, can forgive himself his crash. His lifetime average for entering his garage without incident is still better than .999.

February 17, 1994

A sea change

On an ocean beach last week, I made dinner plans with two tall, tanned lifeguards.

Then they stood me up.

There's not much to say about an event that never happened, except to wonder why a generally happy, self-assured woman like me would let this trivial thing hurt her so.

I travel a lot, alone, to newspaper seminars throughout the country. I easily strike up conversations with the locals. I learn where to shop, where to safely stroll and — most important to me — where to get very good meals.

On my first day, I met Wes. He guarded the beach on which my hotel sat, but mostly he rented out chairs and cabanas. He was tall, and looked down at me from behind wraparound sunglasses. And I guess it must be boring to watch the sea for days on end without much action, because he answered all my questions.

Not just about where to eat, but about how much he makes (minimum $210 a week, plus commission off chair rentals). How it feels to save somebody. And how he fends off high school girls on senior trips, 10,000 of whom paraded on the sand as we spoke in bathing suits I never had the nerve to wear even when I might have.

Wes didn't eat out much. But he mentioned a few places, and I tried one that night.

A mistake. My round-trip cab fare was double the price of my greasy, undistinguished meal.

All I wanted, see, was a small, authentic place with fresh, local fish. A spot the locals keep to themselves, where no tourists go except me.

The next day, when I told Wes of my disappointment, he waved over his buddy Scott, who loves to eat. When he began describing his favorite restaurant, mentioning oysters by name, and describing marinated grilled tuna with sun-dried tomato pesto, I made my proposal:

"Hey! If you guys drive me to this place, I'll buy your dinner! We can start with fresh oysters, and we can talk about the town, and your jobs, and you know, I'm just a journalist who likes to ask questions, and all I really want is some good food and some good talk, and won't it be fun?"

They agreed with gusto. It was gusto, wasn't it? We traded details of our schedules, and swapped phone numbers, and planned to connect the next evening.

I could hardly wait. I felt so pleased to have cooked up this adventure.

But the first number I dialed the next evening went unanswered. The second too.

Finally, I reached Wes at home. "Oh listen!" he said, a little too excitedly. "I forgot to tell you I have a second job, and I forgot I gotta work tonight."

And Scott? "Gee, he didn't mention anything all day. But you can call him at home if you want."

I didn't call him at home.

I closed my eyes and felt pathetic. Is this the tip-off to middle-age? The young find you less appealing than you find yourself, although something in you craves their approval more.

But all I wanted was conversation and a ride! Even with the bribe of dinner, they couldn't spend two hours with me?

That night, I ate at an OK place with a woman from the seminar, a woman about my age, or a little older.

I told her my lifeguard story, of being dismissed by men half my age, laughing and making light of it. I thought I hid my hurt in indifference. But maybe I tried too hard, or maybe she saw something familiar in my face.

Because instead of laughing with me, she sighed, this other woman of a certain age. And then I knew.

May 9, 1995

Divorce's other rift

Everybody worries about the children of divorce, but nobody talks about the friends of divorce.

We are the ones who watch helplessly while those we love split up. We are the ones who contend with grief, guilt, anger and awkwardness from the sidelines.

Like children, we sometimes blame ourselves. Maybe we missed the clues. Maybe we were indifferent to cries for help. Maybe we postponed too long inviting them to the cottage for a weekend alone.

But there are no special support groups for us, no therapists who will urge us to spill out our selfish stew: "Dammit, I liked them! And I liked them together. And I want them back together, because I had such good times with them, and I imagined growing old with them."

Nobody wants to hear our self-centered sadness, because we're adults, and adults are supposed to accept that good things end.

At my age, I ought to have experienced this many times. But I'm going through it for the first time.

We spent more nights in their house than in anyone else's. We ate more meals at their cozy kitchen table, too, and at the big long table he'd carry from the garage on festive summer evenings to set up on the lawn near the pond. He grilled meats or concocted spicy sauces for pasta; she baked bread and pies and cobblers from fresh berries she picked.

Once, in a snowstorm on New Year's Eve, we set off fireworks from the dirt road in front of their house.

The Adirondack chairs we own we bought because they had two we liked. The art on our dining room wall she painted. The cottage we own he owned first.

We talked with them about art and food and family and

ambitions and fears and insecurities and ourselves. Like us, they talked about each other with what sounded like deep affection and good humor. We joked over our lovers' foibles.

Now, it is hard to know what to talk about with either of them. To mention the other's name feels taboo.

She is in the old house but has changed it all around. She's talking about giving one of the dogs — his favorite — away.

He is in an apartment but never cooks there, only sleeps there. It does not feel like home to him. He has not invited us over.

He doesn't know about his dog. And we don't tell him, although we played with that dog since it was a pup.

We can't tell him, because we've heard it's impossible to keep friendship with both halves of a splitting couple if you act as a messenger between them. So we step carefully now in our conversation, as if teetering on rocks in a river.

We watch and evaluate, though. We judge their behavior toward each other, and, against our will, lean from day to day toward one or the other. Is this inevitable? Can we avoid judging? Can we remember that we know only a sliver of the swirl that was their life, and stand quietly on the edge ready to help either one or both?

Tough questions we've asked. Is it really over? Isn't there any hope? No, they insist. But inside we don't believe them. Like children we think, "Maybe we can do something. Maybe if we pray, or wish hard enough, or say the magic word."

We refuse to believe something so old and good broke so suddenly.

We feel foolish for failing to see it cracking.

We want to patch it, them, ourselves, but don't know how.

August 30, 1995

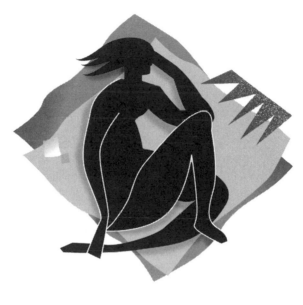

WOMEN

Tears amid the tile

The other day I came upon yet another woman weeping in the ladies' room.

You never know who you will find there, head bent over the sink, splashing cold water into eyes that are gushing hot tears.

You never know when you will hear stifled sobs from behind the gray steel door of one of the stalls. Sometimes it's so pitiful you feel you ought to knock and say, "Pardon me, but can I help?"

Yes, women weep in bathrooms all the time.

That's because in the American workplace, we all roll our eyes and avert our glance from public tears. Then we draw rude conclusions. "Weak," we say to ourselves. "Out of control."

Men, sure, they can stomp and curse. One I know broke his hand punching his fist into a wall. Another kicked wastebaskets and eventually busted a computer with his anger. Men have been acting this way in public for a long time. It used to be rewarded in the workplace, that assertiveness, that drive. It was valuable, for example, on the Ponderosa.

Now we like our working men more sedate, but if they lose it, we excuse them.

Women, mostly, don't holler and swear. Mostly, we cry. And our bosses, our colleagues and even we ourselves are impatient with our tears. Perhaps because tears are so wet and thin, not hard and dry like curses.

That's why many of us women, whenever we feel tears spring to our eyes, half walk, half run to the nearest ladies' room and stay there until we are well again. Often another woman will enter unawares and, without having to be asked, will hold us until we are still.

Well-to-do women stain their silk blouses this way, but no matter.

I don't know what men do to get over their anger.
I don't think anyone holds them.
Too bad for them.
At home, many of us women who are engaged in partnerships weep in the bathroom because it is the most unconditionally loving room in the house. It does not expect us to be a cook, a lover, a hostess or a laundress.

And it's the smallest room in the house. It embraces us. Me, I even leave the light off, sit myself on the shag pink toilet seat cover, and lower my head onto my lap to cry in peace and blissful darkness.

Weeping at the dining room table, or in bed, only provokes conversation. Those with whom we share our lives are sometimes prone to reasoning with us.

But anyone who has ever been in a deep funk — confused and angry and lonely — knows that reason is no balm for the tempests of the soul. It just makes things worse.

So to the weeping room we go.

Some women, especially those in movies, prefer to lock the bathroom door. That's because, especially in the movies, men often want to come in after their women, to rescue them. Such a man will sometimes rap foolishly on a locked bathroom door, cooing his honey's name, cajoling her with simpering reassurances.

What woman would ever choose to leave the comforts of a small, warm, moist bathroom for such a man?

My partner is not like that. He graciously allows me my minutes in the bathroom undisturbed. There, alone, I spill out all my hurt like dirty water from a bucket. And in the breathless heaving that follows, the shattered pieces of my self-esteem can sheepishly regroup.

Men cry too, I'm told, but I'm not sure where. Maybe in the woods, leaning up against the garage, or in the basement at the workbench, or at the bar in their beer.

I think they never cry in bathrooms, though, and I'm glad — because that's our spot.

January 19, 1992

A morel for living

EAST JORDAN — On an ancient hillside covered with spring wildflowers, I walked the other day with a woman who knows the land as well as she knew her husband's hands.

She knows where the elusive and expensive morel mushrooms tend to grow. Her husband taught her how to look, and how to see, and he set a pace for mushroom gathering that used to tire but invigorate her. They would haul pounds and pounds of mushrooms from the woods, once 55 pounds in eight hours.

In 1992, their best year, selling the mushrooms earned them $4,800.

This year, she cannot keep up that pace. But while in similar circumstances I might have spent this spring balled up in bed with the blankets over my head, Edie Bearden is out in the woods hunting for mushrooms because she always has, and because she can count on them.

Walking with Edie, for three hours on a warm and cloudy day, I learn about mushrooms and about living, as we talk together like sisters.

"I'm going out picking every day," she says as we pad through the layers of dead leaves that line the forest floor, "but I'm not finding the millions and zillions that others are this year. I think it's because I'm going to this old familiar place, where I went with John all the time.

"But I come here and I cry. I cry as if I were howling at the moon."

John died last September, on the first night of men's bowling. He sat down at his lane with a Pepsi, raised his hand to his right temple and complained of a headache. Seven hours later he was dead, at 50, of a cerebral hemorrhage.

This would have been her 15th spring hunting mushrooms with him. She was 22 when they married, 37 now.

On his gravestone, in a tiny cemetery a mile from her home, are etchings of a huge buck, and a huge morel mushroom. His stone is almost identical to the one he picked out a year earlier for their 11-year-old son Bradley, who died after accidentally touching a metal tent pole to a high wire in their front yard.

"I wasn't going to function," Edie told me of the months after the two deaths. "I was just going to fade away.

"But then I realized, if you die, or lose your mind, what will happen to your other four children?

"This air is for living people. You have to go on. Doing the laundry and hunting mushrooms and feeding the kids and watching Little League."

She spots our first morel.

"There's one!" she says, with more delight than I expected, pointing to a hollow 10 feet away. All I see are dead leaves and shadows and trillium and the tall droopy greenery of wild leeks, the garlicky aroma of which scents this woods. She walks straight to the mushroom and, with a kitchen paring knife, slices it off. She drops it into a yellow mesh bag that once held potatoes.

She spots others, two, three, four more in the same vicinity. I feel dizzy, trying to see them, too.

"I let my eyes float," she says. "Glancing is best." I hear what she's saying, but I want to stare. I want to work my eyes inch-by-inch over this vast forest floor, convinced if I look hard enough I will see the thousands of mushrooms that must be here, that sell back home in supermarkets for $19 a pound.

Edie knows that's not how it works.

She knows you cannot find every mushroom. She knows you probably miss most of them, leaving them behind to rot. You cannot dawdle, though. You will find more mushrooms if you keep moving, glancing, glancing. You might be tempted to stay under one tree where you've already found three mushrooms, lifting each leaf, scouring the ground for more.

But that would be a mistake. If you linger too long in one place, you will miss the bounty at the next tree, and the next, and over the ridge beyond.

At one ash tree in this huge forest Edie and her youngest children, daughters 8 and 10 years old, found 133 morel mushrooms two days before, counting out loud as they cut them.

When we search the same tree, we find only two. Although hundreds might have sprung up overnight, they did not. But they might, she knows, after we leave.

I work hard to search casually. I try to make my eyes skim the land, not bore into it. I begin to spot mushrooms myself, sometimes in spots

Edie has just covered. She praises me, and I feel excited at so small a thing. I had always thought hunting morel mushrooms required a mysterious intuition and knack, but can see now that anyone, even I, could probably learn it.

In 15 years, it might come easy.

I borrow Edie's knife to slice off a mushroom near its base. The knife is very sharp, and passes through the stem effortlessly, and that which a moment before was attached to the Earth falls into my hand.

I drop it into Edie's bag.

This spring, she picks mushrooms only on these 80 acres she and John bought, although John traveled far and wide to pick morels in secret spots. "Oh, I've been to them with him, but I can't remember quite where they are. And I'd be afraid to go to them, afraid I'd get lost and disoriented, although he never did.

"Here," she says, sweeping her free arm around her, "I don't have any fears. There are no big bad bears. Of course, there aren't in the other woods, either, but in them I don't know where I'm going, or where I've been."

After three hours, the sun is high and the air is hot. I imagine morel mushrooms shriveling up and hiding themselves deeper in the leaves.

My eyes are exhausted. I feel headachy, as I do after searching for Petoskey stones on a pebbly beach, or after reading a difficult book for too long.

The potato bag is half full with hundreds of mushrooms. We've found both black morels, whose season is just ending, and the taller, fatter, white morels, which will last till mid-June. Edie estimates we have about 2½ pounds total, "not bad," she says, "for all the talking we've done." But it's nowhere near the haul she and John might have made on the same land, in springs past.

She gives me half. I insist on paying her, but she refuses, and I relent, taking home a tremendous gift in a brown paper bag.

Five hours' drive south, in my kitchen, I saute the whites and the blacks in separate pans, in real butter, for my husband who, at 53, is exactly as many years older than I as John was older than Edie.

It is late, time for bed, but we eat the mushrooms slowly, and I think about what I've learned and where I've walked with my own husband, and I tell him everything Edie told me about everything she knows.

May 21, 1995

Finance for women

I used to think I could spend my life most honorably if I worked for Planned Parenthood, teaching young women how to use contraceptives to control their destinies.

Now I fear that a bigger lesson, one we've talked about since the '70s, still isn't sinking in: You gotta be able to take care of yourself. Or you risk becoming a prisoner.

In a good world, no woman would stay in a bad situation because she's desperate for someone else's money.

Older women know the value of financial independence. But as a nation we still delude the young. All around us live women weary, bruised and trapped, because someone they counted on turned on them, or left, or died, and they can't make a living wage on their own.

The other day I saw the Tina Turner movie, "What's Love Got to Do With It." Tina's husband beat and insulted her for years, denying her access to the bushels of money they made together. Finally she broke free and is now a rich Hollywood heroine, a role model.

And she's able to say, as she told an interviewer: "I'm not asking any man for money and I never will again."

What powerful words. I thought about battered women and women in dead-end jobs with degrading bosses and women who drive themselves crazy hounding, chasing, cursing and suing men for child-support money. And I thought: "Oh, that those women could sing and strut like Tina. Or do something the world would pay them well for. So they could be free."

Tina's words aren't about men. They're about women, and the too many women who still grow up believing there'll always be someone to lean on.

First, parents provide. Then, a prince rides up with a promise. In exchange for love and money, a woman provides children, dinner, clean folded laundry and emotional support. Oh, and these days she works outside her home, too, but often for a flimsy paycheck, no security and no future.

A neat contract, everybody happy. But we all know what can go wrong.

When I was a teenager, my mother handed me a dime before every date and said, "Call if you need help." That dime was my out. I knew if he got drunk or rude, I always had my dime. It gave me confidence.

Our daughters need skills that serve as that dime did. Hard-world skills that will earn them more money than a Dairy Queen server makes.

Yet the messages the media aim at girls — especially those of whom we expect the least — are intended mostly to help them win men: how to dress, flirt and freshen their lipstick. Useless when the rent is due, the fridge is empty and the kid needs shoes.

We must talk with girls about money more than marriage. We must promote independence more than romance. Maybe we should publish a glossy, pretty magazine called Modern Careers that can compete with Modern Bride.

And when we get wind of a girl who wants to quit school to marry or have a child, we can't smile as if we're happy for her. We have to tell the truth: "You can't afford this choice. Because you can't take care of yourself, or your child. You can't dare remain so vulnerable.

"You don't think so now, but someday you may want to escape. And so far, you have no dime."

July 4, 1993

A girl's World Series

When the Detroit Tigers played the St. Louis Cardinals in the 1968 World Series, I was 14.

Watching each game, I learned about men.

I watched them scratch and spit and rearrange themselves within their pants. TV cameras allowed me my first chance to look at men's bodies up close — bodies that weren't my dad's or my uncles' or the ushers' at church.

I could look at Denny McLain's thighs as he wound up, at an outfielder's forearms as he reached into the air, at a batter's butt as he wriggled into a comfortable stance. In their eyes I saw an unfamiliar and thrilling intensity.

Maybe someday, I thought, a man will look at me that way.

I read every newspaper story and knew every stat. I believed I knew the hearts of these men.

As they stepped up to bat, one after another, I identified those I'd like to kiss. And those I'd like to love.

My hero was Ray Oyler, a scrawny shortstop whose batting average bobbed around .137, but who could snag any ball.

People made fun of him. But I thought I could love him.

The man I wanted to kiss was Bill Freehan, who squatted behind home plate, his face hidden most of the time behind a catcher's mask. Whenever I caught a glimpse of his face I felt the same surge as when I bicycled past my high-school crush's home and, one time out of 100, spotted him in the yard.

Did these men know what they were doing to 13- and 14-year-old girls?

In those days, announcers didn't comment on ballplayers' weight or their hair. I don't remember any stubble. When I roll through the 1968 World Series lineup in my head, I remember how those guys grinned. And I remember how a pitcher in trouble and a batter who struck out at a key moment would hang their heads, exposing the back of their necks.

So vulnerable they seemed. Before I fell asleep each night of the Series, I imagined myself comforting them, holding them, in that weird tangle of motherliness and sexiness that afflicts 14-year-olds, or at least afflicted me.

A friend says her erotic fantasies weren't about ballplayers but cowboys. She imagined "Rawhide's" Rowdy Yates or "Bonanza's" Little Joe as her boyfriend. "I especially liked it when they got hurt, and some woman took care of them," she says. "Isn't that pitiful?"

It seems more old-fashioned than pitiful. Most of us girls felt no longing to ride the range, or play a ballgame in front of millions. We were content to watch, to root, to ache.

Now, 25 years later, Ray Oyler is long dead. Denny McLain is an ex-con and a talk-show host. Bill Freehan is coaching baseball at U-M and is, it turns out, the same age as the man I married.

Watching this year's Series, I sigh. These men are … smaller. Their pants seem too tight. Only Juan Guzman has a face that stirs me. Only Paul Molitor seems like someone with whom I'd want to have lunch.

The men who step up to bat are men I recognize. Men who are slobs, men who are cocky, and men who are decent guys doing the best job they can.

But 14-year-old girls across the nation, I suspect, see more.

I envy them their vision.

October 21, 1993

Empty house, full life

What troubles me each year about Mother's Day is that so many women of substance I've known are not mothers and never will be.

Nobody sends them cards or flowers. Nobody makes them breakfast in bed. Many are never told how much they matter.

Women who bear and/or raise children are to be celebrated: They keep the human race going. The best ones guide and inspire and help their children long after they've outgrown childhood. With any mother other than my own, I'm not sure I'd have the verve I do, or the hunger for adventure, or the courage of my convictions — although we differ on how clean a refrigerator ought to be.

But women who bear nothing more than the usual load of burdens, and raise nothing more than roses, also nurture the human spirit. They rarely get enough credit for it.

They are teachers, doctors, writers, gardeners, engineers, clerks, managers and livers of lives that, despite the suspicions of those who are parents, are not empty or meaningless at all.

When I think back to my childhood, in a neighborhood of identical homes filled with two parents and two or three children, I remember the childless women, too. Watching them, I had the sense that they had to consciously build lives for themselves brick by brick, without the foundation of motherhood on which to rest.

In the corner house on our block lived Helen Dehoney and her husband, Charles. We came to call them Aunt Helen and Uncle Charles. They had no children, and enjoyed a wonderful life of travel and friendships. We'd walk over to sit in their finished basement and eat shrimp — so exotic! so expensive! — and listen to marvelous stories and see slides of distant lands. I don't know what my parents felt during those slide shows, but I thought: "I want to go there, too."

My real Aunt Helen had no children, either, but she loved her dogs and her husbands with gusto, and I still consider her big laugh to be among the world's best. At Polish weddings she dominated the dance floor, her blond hair piled on her head and sprayed stiff. She taught me to polka. She did the cha-cha and other extravagant dances nobody else could do. If she had to, she danced alone.

I liked that. Life's like that.

In high school, my algebra and calculus teacher, Aileen Ryan, never married and had no children. She worked the classroom as if every one of us would someday be a master mathematician, demanding engagement and effort from us, teasing us, criticizing us when we needed it, hugging us when we achieved. I remember her radiant smile, her playfulness, and I remember wondering: "How is it possible that she can seem so happy living in an empty house?"

Time continued to teach me that the customary life formula, the one I grew up in, wasn't the only one.

Now, census data show more women are postponing motherhood, or passing it up, or being denied it. If Hallmark intends to keep making money on Mother's Day, it may want to expand the definition and change the name.

I suggest Mother's and Other Good Women's Day.

May 8, 1994

Anniversary of a suicide

At 4:30 on this morning a year ago, Cheryl Gale got out of the bed where she had slept alone for six years, and padded to the recliner in the living room where her husband, mercifully, had passed a peaceful night.

"Wake up," she whispered, laying her hand on his chest. "I can't stand it anymore."

She offered breakfast, but he wasn't hungry. So she made tea, and they sat in near silence as dawn came and Jack Kevorkian arrived with a machine that ended Hugh Gale's life and began a new one for Cheryl.

She did not expect that police would rope off their home with yellow plastic ribbon and call it a crime scene. Hugh's body sat stiffening in his recliner for 4½ hours before it was removed, while police videotaped him, aiming the camera at his feet, then moving upwards, lingering on his face and the mask through which carbon monoxide had pumped, killing him.

A few weeks ago, Cheryl was enraged to see on NBC's "NOW" news magazine the entire, agonizing 10 seconds of that tape, which she had never before seen.

Nobody's patsy now, Cheryl wrote angry letters to NBC. If nothing else in her life was private anymore, if reporters could stand on her stoop to air their broadcasts, if Kevorkian opponents could toss her trash from the curb into their cars, at least the image of her husband of 22 years dead in his favorite chair should have been hers alone.

Hugh Gale's death was the 13th assisted by Kevorkian, and perhaps the most controversial. At 70, Hugh suffered from congestive heart failure and emphysema, having smoked since he was 14. He was not in pain, but passed out often from lung spasms that cut his air supply. Tubes fed oxygen into his nose 24 hours a day. When he could not walk 10 feet to the bathroom, Cheryl bought him a hand-held urinal.

Before Christmas in 1992, he told Cheryl all he wanted was an appointment with Dr. Kevorkian. But death didn't come easy. Tented in plastic, his oxygen tubes removed, the carbon monoxide mask over his nose, he gasped, "Take it off! Take it off!"

So they waited 15 minutes. Kevorkian offered to come back another day. Hugh smoked a couple of cigarettes to relax. On the second try, he passed out quickly, dying a few minutes later while Cheryl sat in the kitchen, dazed.

Days later, anti-Kevorkian activists produced papers found in the trash that raised questions about Hugh's intent. "Mrs. Gale," a TV reporter asked, thrusting a microphone in her face, "did you kill your husband?"

Now, she says, she would spit at him. Then, hurt and angry, she said nothing.

No charges were ever filed against Cheryl or Kevorkian in Hugh's death.

She is still wary. A woman from the Maury Povich show, impersonating a friend, finagled Cheryl's phone number from her cable TV company. Cheryl bought herself an answering machine after that, screening every call.

For weeks she hauled her trash bags a few doors away to leave on neighbors' curbs. She still burns credit card receipts and personal mail in a coffee can in her backyard.

Friends have been supportive or silent, except for a longtime carpool partner who told Cheryl she hated her for dooming Hugh to hell.

Cheryl's comfort comes mostly from what she calls "our support group" — a half-dozen or so survivors of those who've died with Kevorkian's help.

They meet over lunch or dinner, or for potlucks at the Waterford home of Kevorkian assistant Neal Nicol, who for the next one has offered to cook a turkey if they bring the trimmings.

One weekend, Cheryl joined Sharon Welsh, best friend of suicide No. 3 Sherry Miller, and Cindy Coffey, fiancee of suicide No. 9 Jack Miller, for a weekend up north. When they get together they wear gold chains bearing their numbers.

"I feel like the weak one, that I'm not brave or courageous at all," says Cheryl. "I'm in awe of the other survivors. Yet they feel the same towards me."

She has regained the 14 pounds she lost after Hugh died. Kevorkian brought her bags of hard candies and urged her at least to suck some calories.

Last month, looking for a cake pan in a cupboard, she found boxes of the glass figurines Hugh used in Japanese dish gardens he made. For hours she sat at the kitchen table, unwrapping each one from its tissue, standing them on the table, remembering.

His old gray-and-white sweater still smells like him. When she's blue she hugs it, and imagines him.

His recliner is gone, donated to Salvation Army. She pulled up the old green carpet. On the walls she hung three of Hugh's oil landscapes, of summer, autumn, winter. In a corner curio cabinet his ashes rest in a black cardboard box.

Near the ashes this weekend stood a dozen red-and-yellow tulips, sent by survivor Coffey to comfort Cheryl as the anniversary approached.

Cheryl expected to be at her job as usual today, behind a desk at Blue Cross/Blue Shield. She intended to commemorate Hugh's death instead on Monday night, when a year ago they talked for hours about their ups and downs, and reaffirmed a love which, in Cheryl's case, meant letting him go.

Her plan: to light the white candle from his memorial service. To slide into the VCR the tape of Hugh's conversations with Dr. Kevorkian. To sit cross-legged on the floor, as close to the TV as she can get. And to marvel that one long year is finally over.

February 15, 1994

Means to an end

How does a woman dying of cancer measure her days?
Sandy Davis surveys her home, her two dogs, three cats and
the parrot named Dooley, the man she married 39 years ago when
she was 17, the tax firm they've built, his aging mother who lives
with them, and reminds herself: "I'm needed." That mission, and
the morphine pulsing steadily into her body, keep her going in
these, her last months of life.

At dusk on a snowy Sunday, a beef stew she made for the others
simmers on the stove. She stands at the counter, bent over her own
dinner, the only food she can stomach, a glass of a chocolatey
nutritional drink called Ensure, sipped through a straw. Each eight-
ounce can is 250 calories. She downs five a day, "batting for six."
She has nudged her weight up from 85 pounds to "a high 87."

Chopping carrots for stew is more than routine for Sandy. It is
achievement, "a sense that I can still do things, that my life is not
over."

She credits the morphine.

She was diagnosed with uterine cancer in late 1989, a couple of
months after she quit her 22-year management career at NBD. There
followed surgeries, radiation, a brief sickening round of
chemotherapy and throbbing, dizzying pain as the cancer spread.
One evening, lying on her back on a heating pad, Sandy begged her
husband, Bob: "Put me in a hospital or shoot me in the head. I can't
stand this anymore."

She understood, for the first time, why some have sought relief
with Dr. Kevorkian. But she couldn't. She was needed.

Doctors tried pain-killing patches and pills, but these only
confused her. Her best friend, Virginia Messner, remembers days
when Sandy wouldn't leave her bedroom, couldn't get dressed,
pushed away her friends, lost the gist of simple conversations. "I

watched her slipping away," says Virginia. "I wouldn't have guessed she'd make it to Christmas."

Finally, her doctor told her about Arbor Hospice. "I thought it was a place you went to die," Sandy says. Instead, it meant weekly visitors to her Plymouth home: a social worker, a minister, and a nurse who brings her morphine in a plastic sac and adjusts the pump Sandy wears at her waist in a case the size of a brick, but lighter. "Most women's purses weigh more than this," she jokes, cradling the case as if it were another pet. "Mine used to."

For five or six weeks, she has felt no twinge of pain, not even a headache. She tires easily, catnaps when she can and remains on a 29-pill daily regimen, mostly to counteract morphine's side effects.

If you took an accounting of her life now, here's what you would find:

She has lost her uterus. Her hair. Her appetite, and about 25 pounds. Her stamina, even the ability to carry trash to the garage. Her car, sold last fall. And her faith in a leisurely future.

But she has regained the reassurance of routine. She arises each morning, feeds the animals, selects a wig, gets dressed. She cooks and bakes cookies when she can. At her kitchen table, she works an adding machine to help her husband at tax season.

She watches movies at night, laughing again. And, two weeks ago, Virginia took her to Kroger to shop for food for the first time in eight months.

That tiny excursion felt, she says, remarkably good. "I'm expanding my world." The end is in sight, but she's no longer tumbling toward it headlong, and now dares to hope for one more spring.

January 13, 1993

Postscript: Sandy Davis died April 29, 1993.

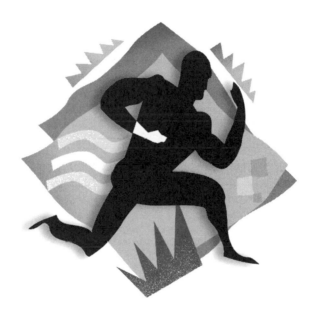

MEN

A marriage smoke screen

Thirty years ago, when they began dating, she didn't care that he smoked.

Nobody cared back then. Cigarettes were cool and cheap and no worse for you than liquor. He didn't smoke as a kid, but once he got a job, he figured out quickly that if you smoked, you could take more breaks.

Within a few years after their marriage, science began affirming what anyone with half a brain knew: Sucking smoke and soot into your lungs all the time dirtied up your innards.

And she started to complain:

"It's no good for you. It will kill you. I don't want to be a widow at the age of 50."

And, "It smells bad. You smell bad. Your clothes smell bad. The whole house smells bad. It's a dirty, disgusting habit that will kill you."

Requests — "I wish you wouldn't smoke in the house" — turned into demands — "Don't smoke that thing in here!"

Finally, "If you're going to be a smoker, I'm leaving you."

What? Sure, he felt dumb for smoking. But how could a bad habit that was once irrelevant turn into grounds for divorce?

To feel better about himself, and forestall her departure, he talked about quitting. All the time. One day a friend challenged him: "Are you serious, or just making conversation?"

"I'm serious!" he insisted, taking another drag.

His friend yanked the cigarette from his mouth. "Then get rid of this."

Chastened, he quit cold turkey. When he told his wife, she said, "Good." But she did not cheer or suggest celebration. What's to celebrate about someone who was once stupid finding some common sense?

For six years, though, the household was happy. Nobody smelled and nobody complained.

Then one night, all the triggers fell into place for him: a dark bar, cold beer, loud music. "What the hell," he thought. "I'll have just one."

You know the rest of the story.

He smoked at his desk and in his car, but never at home. He couldn't smoke at home. He had quit smoking! He was careful never to carry cigarettes or matches or lighters in the vicinity of his wife, although there was other evidence he could not hide.

"Why do you smell like smoke?" she would say.

I was at a bar, he said. Or, I was cooped up in a car with a smoker.

To freshen his breath, he tried marathon toothbrushing, then Hall's menthol eucalyptus drops. Ultimately, he dodged his wife's kisses.

If he had to, he could survive for days without a cigarette, when they were on short vacations, for example. But once he paid a chambermaid to keep his cigarettes and lighter handy so that when his wife took an afternoon nap, or went to the lobby for postcards, he could quickly sneak a smoke.

Over the years, over more than 20 years, many exchanges over this erupted between them.

"Are you smoking?" she would ask, as direct as could be. "No, dammit! Now leave me alone!" he would say. "Then why are you smelly?" "I don't know!" and he'd stomp off.

In retrospect, he says: "It was a game that became necessary to play, or at least a game we chose to play. She knew I was smoking. She had to know! How could she not know? But I denied it. That was our game."

In March, when Michigan voters approved a 50-cent hike in the cigarette tax, he and his shrinking circle of smoking coworkers huddled outside their building complaining, "Where will it end?" He calculated that if he quit, he could give himself the equivalent of an annual $1,000 bonus.

So he stockpiled cigarettes before the tax took effect May 1 and vowed: When they're gone, I'm through.

Eight packs left. Six. Five. He smoked more slowly, stretching a

_____

pack from one day to two.

As his stock shrank, so did his resolve.

When he crushed the last butt, he panicked, prowling the building in search of another cigarette or two to bum. But his smoking buddies were gone for the day.

He stood alone with himself, a man more than half a century old with dirty lungs and a smudgy conscience.

He had no choice. This was it.

He has not smoked since that day, June 5. He does not sneak. He does not stink. He no longer coughs each morning as he used to while his wife wondered out loud if he should see a doctor for his sinuses.

He is thrilled and proud of himself.

He brags about his achievement to anyone who will listen.

Except his wife.

He cannot tell his wife.

But she already knows. She has to know. How can she not know?

October 2, 1994

A line-item treasure

To feel secure, a woman needs four reliable people in her life: A hair cutter. A mechanic. A gynecologist. And a tax preparer.

We must feel safe in their hands. They know things about us we'd rather nobody else know. With them, we ought not to feel stupid or ugly or inept.

I'm lucky. The tax preparer my husband and I use is one of our very favorite people. We actually look forward to passing one evening a year with him.

His name is Tom, but I won't tell you more, because he already has too many clients. Last year Tom turned away a friend of mine, saying: "There's no one I can be sure will treat you as I would, so I can't refer you to anyone, either."

This is not arrogance. This is truth.

Earlier I sent several friends Tom's way. One still mails his stuff to Tom, as if Manhattan had no accountants.

Most of Manhattan's accountants, though, probably don't allow their cats to prowl around while they work. Tom's cat, Fred, was fat and slow and old, but liked to rub up against your legs or sit in your lap while Tom jotted your numbers on forms with a black fine-point felt-tip pen.

Fred died this past year, age 16. Tom told us he cried on his couch for two days straight, as if Fred were a child, and felt a little foolish afterward.

But that's why we like Tom. He's soft, not stiff. He lives alone in a two-bedroom apartment where, in the seven years we've been going there, we've noticed nothing new. Tom's the kind of guy who buys a sofa for life, and it just gets better the more it's used.

In his dining alcove is an old oak table around which he and his clients sit. On the wall above it is an elegantly framed copy of the original 1913 IRS tax form: three pages, plus a page of instructions.

_____

Tom hugs you when you come in the door. He asks about your health. His eyes brighten if you report a new car. If you're driving the same old heap, he commends your thrift.

Tom looks like a hippie Captain Kangaroo with stubble. His hair is long and gray, cut in Prince Valiant style. He wears his flannel shirts unbuttoned half-way down his barrel chest, revealing a sparse population of gray hairs.

This unnerved us at first. Finally I asked him about it. "I feel claustrophobic all buttoned up," he said. His chest hasn't concerned us since. He offers us food and drink when we arrive, tells us to prowl the kitchen until we find something. We have pretzels, or yogurt. One time we brought our own rice cakes. (I was on a diet.)

Usually at least one of us has a Molson Light, but never Tom. He must be sharp. As classical radio music plays in the background, we hand him three-page statements from mutual fund companies, forms peppered with hundreds of numbers, and he frowns and says, "We'll study this," or "This is a terrible form!" We know he will locate the one number we need — "Aha!" — and announce it: "Two-hundred-six-dollars-and-fifty-two cents!"

After two hours, and refills of beer or Pepsi into glasses decorated with cartoon characters, Tom is done. He has filled out every form, speaking aloud each number, rolling his eyes over fine-print rules hidden in big fat books, ranting now and again at how difficult this is, how easy it used to be.

You nod. Tears of gratitude spring to your eyes. Tom is on your side. He shares your values.

With him you are safe.

You hope to God he outlives you.

April 14, 1994

Soft-soap saga

My friend edged into my office the other day, squinting, and said, "You know those plastic soap dispensers you've got all over the house?"

"No," I replied. "I own none. They're dumb. They're a waste of money and plastic, which ends up in landfills. What's wrong," I said, "with an old-fashioned bar of soap?"

He rolled his eyes, including the squinty one, which I noticed looked red and raw. "Well," he said, "I have several of those stupid soap dispensers at home, and here's what happened to me last night with one of them."

This is the story he told:

Naked, about to go to bed, he stood at his bathroom sink to wash his face. He pressed down on the nozzle of the soap dispenser. Nothing came out. He figured the nozzle was clogged with a little dried clot of soap. "Now," he told me, "this is probably a gender thing. A woman would have pulled that little clot out with her fingernail. A smarter man might have, too.

"But I, having failed with brute force, decided my only option was more brute force."

Summoning what force he could, he pounded the flat of his hand against the top of the dispenser. Faster than the blink of an eye, a stream of soap — "a laser beam," he called it — shot from the dispenser straight into his left eye.

I had to interrupt the story at this point for an explanation, since normally dispensers shoot soap down, not up. He told me to imagine turning on a water faucet full blast, then pressing my hand up hard against it, blocking the outflow of water. If I relaxed my hand just a tiny bit, a stream of water would shoot upward. That's what happened with his plastic soap dispenser: He must have loosened the clot blocking the nozzle just a micrometer, forcing the soap stream out in a ferocious blast. I trusted his physics and let him continue with his story.

He couldn't believe the pain. "I felt as if I had been shot in the eye," he said, "or at least poked with a pencil." He wondered for a moment whether his eyeball had popped out and was rolling around on the bathroom countertop. As his nose and his other eye filled with sympathetic mucus, he bounced around the bathroom in pain, banging up against the walls and the towel bars and thinking he must awaken his sleeping wife so she could rush him to an emergency room.

But his tale was too humiliating to tell a physician. Instead, he splashed his face with water. He stumbled to the kitchen, half-blinded, fetched a glass, filled it with lukewarm water and lowered his left eye into it, giving the eye a bath. Finally he stepped into the shower where he stood face up for 45 minutes before he felt well enough to finally crawl pathetically into bed — an hour late.

The next morning, as he told me the story, his eye still looked sorry and bloodshot. Somehow, though, I couldn't help but laugh throughout his tale, and interrupt now and again with what seemed common sense wisdom: "An old-fashioned bar of soap wouldn't have behaved that way."

When he was done, I prodded him: "So what simple lesson did you learn from your unpleasant experience?"

He replied: "That I'll never get any sympathy from you."

February 9, 1995

Is the penis passe?

Men have always harbored secret fears of women.
They have feared women's allure, and women's complex
sexuality, so different from their own. They have feared being
consumed by women, being swallowed whole. They have been
afraid of rejection and of failure.

Mostly, said anthropologist Margaret Mead, "men have always
been afraid that women could get along without them."

So pity the man in America today, more afraid and vulnerable
than ever. Afraid an angry woman will take a hint from Lorena
Bobbitt and slice off his penis. Afraid a woman he works with will
take a hint from Sandra Day O'Connor and haul him to court for a
compliment or a tease.

Afraid that being a man will never be much fun again.

In truth, the penis amputation in Virginia is a symbolic climax to
several decades of shrinking significance for the penis. Decades
during which women have whittled away at the centrality of men
in their lives.

First came an unscientific poll by Ann Landers that revealed
most women would rather cuddle than copulate.

Next came a rash of surveys indicating most women don't have
orgasms during standard intercourse. The penis a man thought was
his most potent sexual tool is tolerated, or even enjoyed. But a great
lover's tools are his words, his hands, his mouth.

Meanwhile, women began choosing motherhood without men.
Some became pregnant with the help of a penis, but others
contracted with a sperm bank, or used semen from a friend,
inserting it with a turkey baster.

Women angry at men chose other women as lovers, or found
sexual pleasure on their own, or did without. Radical feminists
began describing the penis as a weapon, and any act of penetration

as rape.

In San Francisco, a women-owned mail-order company called
Good Vibrations sells four times as many vibrators this year as five
years ago — most, by far, to women. Sex toys give women control
many men aren't willing to surrender. And, said spokeswoman
Laura Miller: "They don't have a lot of the operational problems
penises have."

Ouch.

The American male crosses his legs, chilled by all this and now
by the giddy, guffawing media coverage of the Bobbitts: Quotes
from women who say she should have dropped his penis down a
garbage disposal. Gross generalizations from writers claiming
women are "nearly unanimous" in cheering Lorena's blunt cut.

The average guy is left to wonder if his only noble choice is to
amputate his own penis and turn it in at City Hall, as if it were an
illegal handgun.

But not all of us cheer Lorena, as if this were a football game
with men way ahead on the violence scoreboard. John Bobbitt's
behavior is no credit to any man, but neither is Lorena's any credit
to any woman. Experience has taught most of us how to leave
boorish or dangerous men, then get along just fine without them.

Meanwhile, the world turns: Women with their arms folded over
their chests, men with their legs crossed, hardly anyone feeling safe
or secure, a sorry time for us all.

November 14, 1993

Sympathy for a handsome devil

Why would a very attractive man who could have any woman he wants opt for a prostitute?

Because it's easier that way.

A prostitute who spends 20 minutes with Hugh Grant will not think this is the beginning of something. She will not expect a phone call the next day. She will not tell all her friends, or if she does they will shrug and say, "So? I did (fill in the blank) the other night."

Why would a fellow like Grant, who has a knock-'em-dead live-in girlfriend, say yes to a prostitute?

Probably because he expected something from her he doesn't get from his girlfriend. And he probably got it, or at least the start of it, right before police stepped in to arrest him and the woman, who is 23 and whose name, unlike Grant's, means nothing to anyone.

How can we blame a guy these days?

Especially one who is good-looking, rich and well-known?

The argument that Hugh Grant could have had any woman he wanted is also specious. A lot of women these days don't care so much about looks or money. They want the C-word, commitment, or at least the L-word, love, or, if they're very picky, the S-word: substance.

To seduce a woman like that would have required Grant to heave some pretty heavy lines suggesting he wanted more than mere release from his private tensions.

The other sort of woman, who would have hopped off with him without a second thought, is the one who'd be trouble in the morning. And, even, that night. Even bimbos now want equality in bed. Tit for tat.

Prostitutes don't need seduction. And they expect nothing from you but that you open your wallet.

A prostitute knows her work well.

She is hired to please, and she does whatever is necessary. Often, that's not very much, but it's more than some women are willing to give, no questions asked.

My guess is that whatever was going on in Hugh Grant's white

BMW involved no exchange of dangerous body fluids. I doubt he put himself at risk for AIDS.

If anyone was at risk, it might have been Miss Divine Brown, not the least from trying to maneuver over and around the hump in the middle of those little European cars.

Let's think again about Hugh's girlfriend, model Elizabeth Hurley, and what this prostitute might have had over her.

First, perhaps Divine Brown didn't even know into whose car she was stepping. Maybe she didn't know his name, or any details of his stardom.

Maybe she'd never seen his movies, and didn't know he was the heartthrob of the Western Hemisphere.

She didn't worship at the foot of his fame, or secretly resent it.

Maybe Miss Divine Brown didn't care if he had garlic on his breath, or had had one too many. She didn't care if he hadn't taken a shower since yesterday. She harbored no grudges about some stupid thing he did last week, or last year.

She had no opinions on how he was living his life. He was no more than a man with a longing, no different than a thousand other longings she has encountered, and one she knew she could satisfy.

And maybe he liked that. Maybe he's tired of being a big deal, tired of the limelight and the spotlight and the brown-nosers and the paparazzi and the winking women who think a single shot of themselves on his arm might do them good in the movie business.

Maybe he was tired of his potential.

Maybe he wanted 10 minutes to be a regular animal, of whom no one expected anything. A little like the rich, attractive woman who has sex with the guy who delivers her room-service breakfast. It's neat, clean and over.

No messy implications.

But Hugh Grant got caught. The messiness has begun.

Who knows what he was thinking or feeling or wanting the other night when he invited a 23-year-old stranger into his car. We can guess the nuances are under exploration right this minute, in places more private than his front seat.

All we can know for sure is this:

While the choice Hugh Grant made that night was big news, it wasn't new, nor big, nor one bit surprising when you think about it.

June 30, 1995

No apologies

It remains a mystery to me: Why are so many men so stingy with "I'm sorry"?

Men may think they're apologizing. But we hardly know it from the way they stall and muddy their apologies with extraneous words.

Last fall, for example, Henry Kissinger apologized for wiretapping the home phone of a White House aide 23 years ago. After a 19-year lawsuit forced him to, Kissinger said, "It is something if circumstances were repeated, I would not do again."

He wouldn't say "I'm sorry."

I wasn't surprised.

Those are women's words.

Last week, state senators Gil DiNello and Jack Welborn had a chance to redeem men in the apology arena. They blew it.

A woman reporter had overheard them joking about what one called "the titty bill," a bill to ban nude dancing. She felt offended by their language and wrote a column about it.

Both men might have stood the next day in the Senate to say "I'm sorry." Or, if they wanted to be wordy, "I'm sorry my language offended."

Instead, one senator refused to apologize unless the reporter insisted the remarks were directed at her. The other accused her of being obsessed with political correctness and said she needed to grow up. Then he demanded an apology from a woman senator who had sided with the reporter.

What a mess.

"I'm sorry" would have ended the story.

Granted, some of us women overuse the words. We'll apologize for anything. We say "I'm sorry" for a cantaloupe that turned out not quite ripe. For a kid who's misbehaving. For a contrary opinion.

For feeling sick, or looking tired. Even for an unpleasant bit of news we must deliver: "I'm sorry, but the party store was out of honey-roasted peanuts."

Women have also discovered that it's easier to say "I'm sorry" in the middle of an argument than to carry it on forever. Sometimes we apologize when we only half mean it but want the fight to end so we can go take a shower and drink a bourbon in peace before bed.

Is this healthy? Hardly.

But it's healthier than male resistance to timely, neat apology. Men seem more at ease explaining, justifying, dancing around and defending themselves.

Their apologies are grudging. They rarely say, "You're right. I screwed up. I'm sorry."

Male friends insist I'm wrong. But only one could cite an instance when he had quickly and cleanly apologized to a woman. He complained, "I was looking for forgiveness, or at least understanding, but instead I got more of a lecture."

That's too bad. Maybe men don't apologize because women make it so hard. Everyone should take "I'm sorry" at face value — especially because those words are an achievement for a man. If we beat up a man afterward, he may never say "I'm sorry" again.

Maybe "I'm sorry" humiliates him. Maybe he flashes back to being slapped on the bottom by Mama.

Or maybe he loses points in the great game of life by conceding a mistake. Maybe he's stalling, hoping his opponent will give up. Or apologize first.

That's what women do. We know the longer we wait for an apology, the more apology we'll need to satisfy us. And the more we insist on apology — "You know you were wrong. Now just say it!" — the more men resist.

"I'm sorry" comes easily from men's lips only after they step accidentally on our feet in elevators.

And even then, they might just say "Oops."

May 3, 1993

In praise of older men

Regrets, I've had a few, but always with men who knew no more about life than I did and were just as baffled about what to say in a receiving line.

One man, just two years younger than I, had the fantasy life of a 12-year-old. He dreamed of making millions as a combination architect/hypnotist/magician. As my mother had taught me, I listened intently to his plans, looked into his eyes, nodded appropriately, and asked challenging but not discouraging questions. I was very fond of him and tried to believe in his dreams, but I couldn't.

He is still poor.

Another younger man considered it entirely appropriate to exit from a movie with no opinions about it. Nothing to say about the plot, the characters, the moviemakers, or even about a Hollywood that would allow such a movie to be made. Nothing to say about anything.

Still another — several years younger — loved to drink beer and have dusk-to-dawn conversations. When light began to creep up the edge of the sky, we found mugs of coffee and fried eggs at an all-night place, then stumbled away to our offices.

Young men have a few assets: They have stamina on the dance floor. They have wild dreams that can keep your own flagging interest in life afloat. They have thick hair, and can easily read road maps. Usually, they don't require afternoon naps. But chances are you will have to live with them through the extraction of their wisdom teeth, not a pleasant episode, and the eviscerating of their dreams, likewise gruesome.

Older men have already lost their wisdom teeth and their illusions. They have more wounds, but they also have more scars, and that makes them tougher. Older men know more than younger men, as a newspaper with more pages contains more information. They know what to say at funerals. They know how to issue sincere compliments to babies and elderly women. They keep track of the time, and realize, from experience, that staying up too late ruins the next day.

They prefer mornings to nights.

My favorite older man, 13 years my senior, is simpatico with my own rhythm. We go to bed at the same hour, but he rises earlier than I, making the tea and fetching the newspaper from the porch. Sometimes, he awakens as early as 4:30 a.m., to the sound of the newspaper against the stoop, then lies awake thinking. But he does not fret about the stock market, or the latest dent in his fender, or wonder what his tie might say about him at his important meeting that day. Instead, he muses about what is left of his life, and how he can make the most of it. Not the most money, but the most meaning.

Older men worry about making a difference in the world. So do younger men, but younger men tend to push those frets away, postponing them for later. Older men worry there may not be much more later, which is why even if they long for a midday nap, they hesitate to take one.

Older men understand delight. They know it is a sly thing. More than anyone, they understand that ragtag aphorism about letting happiness land on you, like a butterfly, instead of chasing after it. Most older men have chased pleasure plenty in their lives, ending up exhausted and with only so much happiness as they could clasp in their two fists. Older now, they chase it less. Instead, when delight alights on them, they remain perfectly still so it stays as long as it can.

Older men have slow hands. They know how to touch. They know the pleasure is in the desire, not the climax. They do not itch to keep score. They know that one week they will win, and another they will lose, but over the course of a year, or a decade, or a marriage, things tend to even out.

Because of that, they do not weigh their days, measuring them as successes or failures. They do not get worked up if you are too tired to even snuggle. They do not count the day lost if their favorite coffee shop is closed for remodeling, or their boss humiliates them, or they find themselves immobilized on a freeway for three hours.

This is unbelievable to those impatient youngsters among us, who count a vacation a failure if it rains five days out of seven. But living with an older man gives a younger woman an edge in learning the things that only experience teaches.

Older men have come to realize that people are more important than things, that love is more rewarding than power, that children are more loyal than corporations and that time is pitifully short. I carry in my wallet a scrap of paper from a fortune cookie. "A lost inch of gold may be found," it says, "a lost inch of time, never." I'm sure it was written by an older man.

Older men not only know wise things, they know old things. They can hum the best dance tunes. They can quote the lines from great old movies you never heard of. They can explain many of the moments you chose to forget from high school history classes, being too young and stupid and self-involved.

They also remember the way things used to be between men and women — the unspoken contracts, the hidden feelings, the rules for proper behavior, public and private. Many of them, including the man I live with, are glad for the new ways. Younger men don't realize things were ever any different.

Certainly there are practical reasons to love an older man. You need not worry about whether you'll still love him when he has lost his boyish good looks, for one. For another, you will be able to dip into your IRA when he turns 59, without waiting until you are. Plus, if you plan things right, you can both retire long before you would have been able to if you were alone, or with a younger man. Even if you don't retire, all those senior citizen discounts will apply.

But the very best thing about older men is that they appreciate older things, and appreciate them more the older those things get — wine, cheese, books, friends. As you grow older, they will appreciate you, too, although you will always be "a younger woman," for whatever that's worth.

I moved 2,500 miles to live with the older man I love after another older man — perhaps 25 years my senior — gave me some advice. I met Ed Orloff, a San Francisco editor, very close to the end of his life. We had only about six hours of conversation, over three meetings, as he was dying of Lou Gehrig's disease. We sat in his yard and talked about my work and his and the state of journalism in America. We shared chocolate almond ice cream. He invited me to pick kumquats from his trees.

One evening at dusk he asked me who my best friends were, and I told him about Larry. He asked why we were so far apart. I told him I wasn't sure I wanted to pull up my roots, quit a very good job, and leave everything behind for a man.

"But do you love him?" he asked me, his voice raspy and gravelly from the disease that ultimately would silence him. "Yes, I do," I said, "but …"

He interrupted me, shaking his head, his hands gripping the arms of his wheelchair. "We've got only one shot at this," he rasped. "One shot."

I got the message. I left San Francisco for Larry, and for Ed, whose wisdom I trusted.

August 6, 1989

Daughter's love comes first

H is church may punish him. If they ask him to repent, David Hines will refuse.

He loves his daughter, and now, finally, she has found happiness. So on Saturday, he will preside over a ceremony in which she will commit herself for life to the woman she loves.

"I can't understand the physiology, because it's foreign to me," says Hines. "But I understand the love. And the love is the same."

Hines is a minister and elder of the Reorganized Church of Jesus Christ of Latter-Day Saints, a church, like most others in America, that does not condone homosexual behavior, let alone bless the unions of gays and lesbians.

Before he learned his daughter Elaine was lesbian, he stood with his church in opposing homosexuality.

Now, he stands with her.

"When it happens to you," he says, "you have to make choices, immediately. And my God, I could not choose against her.

"I have come to believe that God would not create people one way, then condemn them for it."

Elaine told her parents she was lesbian eight years ago, although her mother had suspected since Elaine was a little girl. At first, her father could hardly accept it, although he never said a reproachful word.

But in twice-weekly phone calls between her home in Kansas City and theirs in the Upper Peninsula, Elaine talked to her parents about her life, and answered their timid questions. She had always seemed such a troubled and depressed teenager, so they felt relief as she seemed to be finding peace.

When she moved in with Dee Carver last fall, David Hines recognized that she was happier than ever. So how could he refuse when she asked him to lead their commitment ceremony?

"I have come to the position where I am," Hines says, "because I love her, because she is very important to me, and I was forced to accept it. Forced by love."

On Wednesday at dawn, he and his wife, Joan, climbed into their pickup truck for the two-day drive south. Their land was springing to life, as it reliably had for centuries, the earth covered with trilliums and trout lilies.

In Kansas City, though, any old reliable definitions of family won't apply. The day after the ceremony, the Hineses will celebrate the 47th anniversary of their own marriage at a fancy dinner with Elaine and Dee, with an unmarried son and with another son and his wife, who have separated but still get along.

"It's just different," Hines says of his family, laughing as a man who is flexible and wise will do.

About 150 friends will surround Elaine and Dee at the Saturday afternoon ceremony. Elaine wrote the brief vows, which deliberately don't mention God or include any of the well-worn language of standard marriages. Privately, Elaine and Dee call the ceremony a wedding, but they don't want anyone else to think they're pretending to get married.

They know they cannot, legally or religiously. So their vows speak simply of honesty, fidelity and nurturing.

Both women will wear linen — Elaine a pink suit, Dee off-white slacks with a matching silk blouse and pink cardigan. They will exchange plain gold bands.

Finally, Elaine's father, in his special gray church suit, will present them to the crowd and say, in words Elaine asked him to, "May the Universe forever smile upon Dee and Elaine."

But Hines, thinking it over from the woods of the UP, has decided he will and must say more. At the very end he will dare, as if Elaine and Dee were marrying, to ask the blessing of the Lord upon this couple and their love. The same love which anchors any union and any family, no matter its shape.

May 21, 1993

It's a dirty job

Our new Ranger truck really stank the other day, like a sackful of old garbage.

It didn't take long to figure out the problem. A small bird, no match for the truck on a country road a few days earlier, now was decomposing somewhere in its innards.

My husband was out of town. This problem was all mine.

I sprayed the grille with a long hard blast of water, but nothing plopped onto the pavement.

Now what?

Put up with it, I told myself. Hold your nose. Eventually, I figured, it would fall out or biodegrade. But no way would I poke around in there to goose it.

That afternoon, on my way to visit my in-laws, I aimed for potholes, hoping to dislodge my dead companion. When I arrived, I casually mentioned my predicament: "Gee, that soup you're cooking sure smells good. Speaking of smell …"

Lo, my father-in-law leapt to his feet. He grabbed a long-handled barbecue fork and went to work on the carcass in the radiator, while my mother-in-law and I stood 20 feet away and grimaced.

I marveled at this. At 78, he had not hesitated to take on a nasty job, one I wouldn't touch.

Was I seeing sheer macho? Gallantry? Or duty, with nausea its price?

What about me? A fair-weather feminist, all for equal opportunity except when the job is ugly. Then I'm happy to let men do it.

One woman I know cleans her household's toilets but won't empty its cat litter. Her husband does. Others won't touch huge hairy insects they find perched on the edge of the bathroom sink. Guess who kills them?

These are tiny unpleasantries men take on. Others include cornering bats and burying deceased pets.

Of course, women who are alone acquire the nerve to do these things themselves — or hire men for the job. And one could argue that women in relationships take on plenty of yucky duties involving childbirth, child care and the disposal of leftovers forgotten in the back of the fridge.

But men rarely refuse the bigger, more dangerous assignments. Women have let men do the nation's fighting and killing for centuries. Now there's talk of allowing women to volunteer for combat. Don't expect a stampede.

Off the battlefield, too, we shrink back.

When something goes bump in the night, I wake up and gasp. "What's that?" But he is the one who crawls out of our bed to investigate. I never ask him to. He just goes, while I pull the covers over my head, terrified that he will be blown to bits by a burglar.

What would happen if, in the middle of the night, we woke to a noise and he trembled and whispered, "I'm so scared. Sweetie, can you go look?"

I can't imagine.

Don't men gag at the prospect of a maggoty bird? Don't they suffer midnight dread of dying in their jammies in the hallway?

Sure, they say. But it has to be done. And someone has to do it.

But why them and not me?

A few weeks ago, on vacation in Bermuda, my husband and I rented a tiny scooter, the only vehicle available to tourists. "Will you be driving at all?" the scooter instructor asked me. I blanched.

So the man I love drove the wobbly thing all week on twisty, traffic-packed roads, me hunched behind him, my arms around his belly. When we left Bermuda, the muscles in his back were tighter than when we arrived.

He might have refused to drive. If he had, I might have swallowed my fear and piloted the thing. Or we'd have walked.

He didn't refuse, though. So I let him. But every night I rubbed his neck.

November 9, 1992

A march of meaning

The TV images were stunning: masses of black men, standing shoulder to shoulder. Not pressing desperately forward for job interviews. Not milling in anger, ready to throw bricks. Not shuffling in indifference or bewilderment at life's everyday demands.

If you watched, you saw a man with his hand on the shoulder of his 8-year-old nephew, whose father worked overtime Monday as a Washington, D.C., police officer. You heard this small boy say he was learning about unity, love and people taking care of one another, things every child should learn.

You saw men in the sun, in white shirts and T-shirts, in kente cloth caps and baseball caps, pumping the air with their fists in time to music made for them by other black men.

You saw black men spanning five generations, standing side by side with their ancestry and their progeny. Some men wept. Strangers embraced strangers, and why? Because they shared enough life experience to know they belonged in the same spot for one day.

Columnists and social commentators didn't catch the significance of the Million Man March until about 10 days ago, but then many of them lit into it and its originator, Louis Farrakhan. A minister of hate, they called Farrakhan, a man who would lure black men together into a swamp of hate.

Some women groused about being left out — women who for years have spoken bitterly about the failures of the men they've tried to love.

Everybody who has ever complained about the Black Man in America — his shiftlessness, his violence, his unreliability — complained about this march. With all the ugly, vile and hopeless things in the world to deride, I wonder why cynics work so hard to poke holes in efforts that aim high and might well float.

Critics, some black, spoke of this event as if every black man who traveled 12 hours on a bus, hunching for sleep on a small hard seat, would fall sway to Farrakhan's separatist philosophies. As if these men were too stupid to think for themselves. As if they weren't coming with their own personal agendas, many too private to be voiced.

This many men do not travel so far for hate.

Only hope lures people like this. Hope and hunger.

From the stew of messages that spilled from the stage in Washington, each man picked the words he hungered for, casually shoving aside the rest. No big deal. We all do that every time we listen to a flamboyant minister or politician.

One black man, a 53-year-old fisherman, flew from Fairbanks, Alaska, to Seattle, then rode the train for three days. Imagine what he will carry back on the train, in his head and his heart.

If only we could listen in on conversations on buses and trains as they carry hundreds of thousands of black men back home today. President Clinton encouraged a dialogue Monday in a speech in Texas.

He called on every important person and every average person, too, to "take personal responsibility for reaching out to people of different races, for taking time to sit down and talk through this issue, to have the courage to speak honestly and frankly, and then to have the discipline to listen quietly, with an open mind and an open heart."

It sounds so small. But let's not underestimate the power of even one day's images and words to stir human beings.

This is how change begins.

October 17, 1995

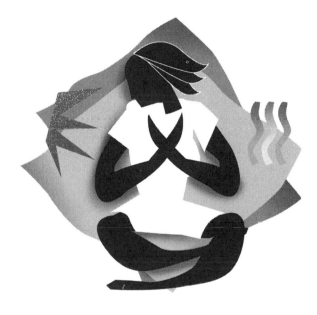

AT HEART

A hand for the roller rink

When we were 13 and growing up in the '60s as good Catholic girls, few opportunities existed to touch boys without shame. That's why we loved the roller rink.

Most of us, intimidated by our sexual stirrings, were not so bold as to approach a boy for affection on, say, the sidewalk in front of church after mass.

The roller rink provided excuses.

We sat on wooden benches lacing up our skates, whispering to each other, watching the boys on other benches lacing theirs.

We stepped onto the old wooden floor of the rink, scratched and worn by thousands of skaters before us. We swung our arms and our legs moved, and suddenly we were flying! Moving faster than we would have thought possible, pushed to skate even faster by those bearing down on us from behind.

We teetered, dizzy. With one eye we watched as the boys we liked caught up with us, and then, so as not to spin out and fall, we reached out to them.

They reached out to us.

And for a few moments, we skated hand in hand.

Our hearts pounded. Our faces burned. We pretended nonchalance. "Thanks," we gasped.

Then we or they let go without a word and skated away, and that was that.

What did the boys think afterward? Did they think anything? Did they replay that touch as we girls did, circling the rink, torturing ourselves with analysis? "Am I right that he held my hand much longer than he might have? And tighter, too? I think his hand was even sweaty! Do I dare hope he might take my hand again? Would that be pushing things? Why won't he look at me now? Is he embarrassed? Did I make a mistake? Can I dare look him in the eye again?"

Repressed memories of those pitifully anguished touches washed over me the other day when I heard that our roller rink, the Rollerdome on Warren at Outer Drive in Dearborn Heights, had burned to the ground. I couldn't remember the color of the walls, or the music that played, or the cost of the skates, or anything but the way we spent the whole evening watching the boys we liked best, looking for clues, waiting for chances.

Afterward, we stumbled into the warm spring night and climbed sweaty onto the bus — these were church teen club outings — and fervently hoped the bus driver would leave the lights out. No one ever necked on the bus. But if the lights were out, and if you chose a seat a few seats behind the boy you liked best, you could watch his silhouette in the streetlights, and imagine kissing him.

We used to take that bus to the Boblo docks, too. We knew the spots on the boat where you could stand alone with a boy and gaze down at the water and talk about fish and accidentally brush shoulders.

The ride home from Boblo, if the lights were out, lasted a delicious hour.

Boblo is closed now. The roller rink is ashes. They say 13-year-olds are different now, too, that they're not thrilled anymore by the mere touch of a boy's hand, or a glimpse of his profile in shadow.

I'd rather not believe that. I'd rather believe some things never change, and that some kids will miss the roller rink as much as we sentimental adults will.

April 21, 1994

Love makes you fat

My friend's neck is thicker than it used to be. His belly, always flat, now billows just a bit.

He's only 29, but he's in love.

And love makes you fat.

My friend used to think he was in love quite often, but I knew he wasn't because he was still starving himself. When you're worried about a little fold of skin above your belly button, you're not in love yet. You're still in lust. Or infatuation.

If you can't relax about your body, you're not relaxed about yourself. You're not sure the other loves you. You worry he or she might leave for someone thinner.

Romance makes you thin, but love makes you fat.

When you're really in love, you trust that you'll be together for quite some time. The foods you rejected trying to look your best now serve to grease your conversations and your days.

You greet each morning with joy, and celebrate with eggs and sausage and fresh-squeezed orange juice and slabs of bread oozing with butter and jam.

At lunch, you're so busy telling all your friends about your new life that you hardly notice how much you shove in your face while you're talking.

At dinner, you want to linger. You sit together at table, telling the tales of your lives, picking at platters of food that ought long ago to have been removed to the kitchen counter. Maybe you drink wine, too. It doesn't matter because probably you won't do anything else this evening except eat and talk and drink wine and then go to bed, where your activity will make you feel fit.

It's when you lie in bed alone, squeezing the flesh of your belly between your own fingers, that you feel most fat. The same body in bed with someone you love, who loves you back, feels somehow thinner.

I think of a variation on that old saying about sex and love: If a couple puts a nickel in a pot for every calorie shunned in the first year, and takes one out for every calorie shunned thereafter, many nickels would remain in the pot.

My friend, for example, tells of a shopping excursion for dinner with the man he just moved in with. He has in mind a low-fat pasta dish and a small green salad. But doesn't that fresh mozzarella look good? Wouldn't it be a splendid salad with tomato and basil and olive oil? And maybe instead of a limp fresh tomato sauce, wouldn't a pesto be heartier and tastier and more satisfying on a winter's night?

It's easy to get carried away. A pint of Ben & Jerry's Cherry Garcia frozen yogurt would be perfect in bed. A pint of amaretto to spike the coffee would be great, too, with a few squirts of whipped cream on top.

When you're in love you feel larger inside. All that space needs to be filled. Steamed green beans don't fill it.

I would never suggest that only love makes you fat. We all know that loneliness and fear and, OK, hormone disorders will make you fat, too.

But love fat is special. It's noble. It's right. It's good. It's something to celebrate and even show off. It tells the world you're at peace and at ease, and understand what's important in life. Because as longtime lovers know, and as Garrison Keillor put so well, "Sex is good, but not as good as fresh sweet corn." With butter, together, at table.

February 13, 1994

Once-a-year love

Every year about this time, when the Earth is lush with summer, a man places a call to the office of a woman he has known for 40 years and, with trepidation, asks if she might join him again for a picnic.

They meet once a year, no more, for half an afternoon between noon and 3 at a picnic table near the Huron River. They meet to commemorate her birthday, and have been meeting this way for seven or eight years.

This year she turned 53. He is 58. Each has been been married for more than two decades, but not to each other, although he would have liked that, because she is the love of his life.

He never says it in quite those words, but they both know it. Every year he tells her she is beautiful, even if she has gained 20 or 30 pounds. He reminds her what a fine human being she is, and it's surprising how much she needs to hear that.

She is a woman of high professional achievement, but she rarely hears words as ripe with emotion as his. Her husband, whom she loves very much, is a reserved man who, for her birthday, might give her a card and underline a word or two.

I will call them Allison and Lloyd because, while her family knows and respects that she reserves one day a year for Lloyd, and even teases her gently about it, his wife does not know about his annual picnics, although she has heard Allison's name.

Nothing clinically sinful ever happens on these outings. They talk heart to heart, and split a couple of sandwiches, and finish off a bottle of wine and show off pictures of their kids. Sometimes they walk through the woods, or she kicks off her shoes to dangle her feet in the cool river while he watches, shoes and socks on, smiling at everything she is.

Lloyd thinks no loving God could possibly deny him a three-hour picnic with a woman he has loved for so long. Allison is like a polished stone he keeps in the pocket of his heart.

He doesn't want to pull it out and analyze it.

He never calls or writes to her in between their picnics. He knows her boundaries, and his own, although in his subconscious, which he cannot control, she is always present. Even as the minutes of their picnic tick by, Lloyd never asks for more time. He is a man of strict routine and habit, and his family expects him home at the same hour each afternoon. When they part, when she drops him back at his workplace, before he steps out onto the sidewalk, he leans over and kisses her. For a few seconds, their lips touch.

And that is all.

That is enough.

She doesn't remember the day they met but he, of course, does. He was a senior in high school in the mid-Michigan town where they both grew up. She was 13 and had been invited to his English class to read her poetry aloud. He can still see her: "She wore a blue calico dress with a black patent leather belt, and her hair was cut in a Prince Valiant style, that lovely black thick hair of hers. That set all my emotion in motion."

As they grew a bit older they went out some, usually in groups, but sometimes alone. He was never as central in her life as she was in his, and they both knew that. She was outgoing and gregarious and daring and witty, and he was shy and timid and unsure of himself.

"Her assets are a litany of my weaknesses," he says. "I never even wanted to be No. 1, but she has always been No. 1. I am funny only because I am not funny."

Each went on to marry someone else, she a tall and strapping man of few words, he a woman who would have him, a good and kind woman but no one as stirring as Allison. Allison did not invite him to her wedding — "I think it would have hurt him too much" — but he sent her a gift, a pepper grinder she still uses.

Over the years her life expanded. She had three children, and earned five degrees, and took on bigger challenges at work, and learned to feel at ease speaking to hundreds or talking intimately to one person over lunch, charming them with her stories and her laughter and her zest.

He, meanwhile, deliberately shrank his life down. He quit a stressful job for an easier one, and kept to himself at work, arriving and leaving at the same time each day. Having fun was hard work for him. Laughing was rare. But when he remembered Allison, he remembered how fun and laughter felt.

He kept track of her as she moved about the country, and kept note of her birthday on his calendar.

A decade ago, when he and his family landed in a spot near her town, he summoned his courage to call and ask if they might have lunch. The first time they ate in a Holiday Inn dining room where he felt edgy and watched.

In the following year he scouted out parks, and found an isolated place where he would not be distracted by joggers or other picnickers from the beauty of her face, and the pleasure of her company.

They have met there ever since.

This year, as usual, Lloyd called her office in early June. As usual, he told her it had taken him almost a year to summon the nerve.

As usual, that made her smile. What's he afraid of? That she will say no?

That is exactly what he fears, that he will shrink in significance and fall off the chart of her life. So he asks her for very little, and enjoys it enormously. "It is precious time," he says. "And will I dream about her every night for the next six months? I might for the next year, yes."

They picked last Monday to meet, a few days past her birthday, but the only time they could manage. She told him when he called that she was being courted for a bigger job, 1,500 miles away, and flying back and forth for interviews.

He got up at his usual time on Monday, just before 5 a.m., and gathered the props for the picnic: The red-and-white checked tablecloth he bought special for it many years ago, and which he keeps on the bottom of a pile in the linen closet. Two tulip-shaped wine glasses. A corkscrew. A cooler. Together with a glass vase from work, which he fills with wildflowers, the props help make a perfect stage, he thinks. "It's almost like 'Casablanca,' like a romantic little cafe along the Huron River."

But on this Monday he felt a little discombobulated, pretending, too, that maybe she wouldn't leave, refusing to think this might be their last picnic.

By the time he got to work he realized he had left all the props in his room in the basement. So he had to improvise: borrowing a cooler and some water glasses from work, buying a cheap corkscrew and a blue paper tablecloth.

Worse, the park where they normally meet was closed for maintenance. They had to go someplace else, where joggers kept coming by and where the view was different, and even the air. Not dry, crisp and bright, as in the past, but this time sodden with humidity, threatening rain.

As they settled opposite each other on the rough benches of a picnic table, though, it was as if they had picnicked just last week. He asked about her sister, and she showed him a beautiful new picture of her daughter, and she told outrageous stories about herself, and he found himself laughing.

And when she told him about the job she might take, halfway across the country, he teased her about sneaking away for the weekend this time next year, and spending three days with her, instead of just three hours.

They both knew he'd never do it. If anything, he might place a birthday phone call, or send a birthday note.

She thought: "If these picnics end, I think I'm going to feel like I finally got old." And she thought: "Everybody needs a Lloyd in their lives," and felt herself swell with gratitude that Lloyd had stuck with her.

They finished the bottle of cabernet. She drank most of it, and what he did drink made him feel a little tipsy, a little out of control.

The sky darkened as they gathered up the props. As usual, she kept the wildflowers to take home. They tossed out the sandwich wrappings and the wine bottle and, this year, the tablecloth, too.

When they got into the car, though, and she turned the key to start it, he broke the routine. He said something he had never said before. He said, "Turn it off for a while," and she complied.

He leaned toward her and put his hand behind her neck and pulled her face toward him and kissed her. Kissing her while they were still in the park, a full 10 minutes before their time was over, was not in the usual order of things. But at that moment, there was nothing he wanted to do more.

Startled, teetering on the edge of her emotions, she said something dumb: "Please don't do anything either of us would regret." As if Lloyd ever would.

"I'm really going to miss you," he told her, looking into her eyes and seeing, despite her age and her success, a pretty 13-year-old girl reading poetry in a calico dress.

Then as he settled back in his seat, she started the car again, and dropped him back at his work where they kissed once more, this time in the usual spot. Within 15 minutes each was on a different road home, as the clouds released their rain.

July 2, 1995

'Yes' will thaw the freeze

Steve hopes Joy will marry him.
He hung a banner from an M-14 freeway overpass last week to pose the question: "Marry me, Joy? Steve." It was the second freeway proposal I'd seen in a week.

I don't know Steve or Joy, nor do I remember the names of the other couple, but I have advice for them:

Go for it. And go for it quickly.

November is upon us, and winter has already snuck its cold, clammy hand down our shirts, and there are only so many ways to get through the next few months, love being one of the best.

The nights are lengthening like shadows now: On Monday, Nov. 1, we had 1 hour and 24 minutes less daylight than on Oct. 1. You drive home in the dark and, as the days dwindle down for another 7½ weeks, soon you'll drive to work in the dark, too.

You'll eat breakfast and dinner in the dark and when you look outside, all you will see is your own wan face reflected in the glass.

Your best intentions regarding waterproof boots and serious gloves and hats won't matter. Winter will turn you wet and cold and dispirited.

But a spouse can light a fire before you get home.

A spouse can pare a few apples and start applesauce simmering on the stove.

In bed, a spouse is someone against whose body you can warm your feet.

On mornings when you're sniffly, a spouse might start your car 10 minutes before you climb into it. A spouse might scrape the ice from the windshield.

Not that marriage is the only answer to winter.

Plenty of companions with whom you aren't legally paired can help ease the weight of winter, including dogs. But in marriage exists the illusion of a bit more security, in the same way that two cords of wood neatly stacked in the garage give the illusion of warmth all winter.

The wood might prove green. Or the winter may be so brutal that the wood burns away more quickly than you expected. The wood, and the love, may be gone by April.

But to have them in November is comforting.

A few weeks ago in North Dakota I met a woman, 43 years old, who had just married the man with whom she had lived for 12 years. Twelve years! I was bewildered. "It just seemed the right time," she shrugged. And, she said, her husband believed he could win a high-ranking job more easily if he could honestly report he was married, and not just shacking up like an aging hippie.

But her explanations seemed inadequate. I wondered if after 12 years of prairie winters, they hadn't seen November descending like a slab of concrete, and decided this time they wanted a woodpile.

It's your choice, Steve and Joy. People who live alone survive winter quite handily, what with leaded coffee and bean soup and good books and furry dogs. But if solitude is what you choose, Joy, and what you end up with, Steve, I've got a bit more advice:

Never eat out of the pot in November. Never eat standing up. Find a nice bowl and light a little candle and sit down in front of it and eat slowly.

The winter will be long.

November 2, 1993

A schoolgirl's crush revived

Pushing an empty shopping cart toward the supermarket the other night, I looked up from the slush and saw the face of Kevin Gregor.

He was my first serious crush, and I hadn't thought about him in decades. We were in third grade. He was the cutest boy in class, all of us girls agreed.

But he was aloof, too. Stuck-up, we called him. We figured he knew exactly how cute he was.

He intimidated me. I could say nothing more to him than a timid "Hi." Sometimes he'd say "Hi" in return, and I'd memorize the sound of his voice speaking that word, and replay it over and over again.

Once, our teacher asked him and me to stay after school to clean the chalkboards. I remember him pulling over chairs for us to stand on. I remember trembling as we ran our erasers up and down, silently, side by side.

In the slush outside the supermarket the other evening, Kevin Gregor's name flashed into my head as I looked into the eyes of a 40-ish man, graying, weary, pushing a full cart out of the store I was about to enter.

Our shopping carts passed in the night.

I did not speak. He did not stop.

And that was the end of it.

"Why didn't you ask him if he was Kevin Gregor?" a friend shouted at me over lunch a few days later.

"Because he probably wasn't!" I protested.

But he might have been. Which might have been worse.

What would I have said?

"When you were 8, I thought you were really cute."

Or: "I think it's because you were so stuck-up in the third grade that I am still irrationally attracted to arrogant men."

All scripts seemed foolish. There's no way I could have emerged from any encounter with the purported Kevin Gregor without feeling like an awkward third-grader again.

The Kevin Gregor sighting unnerved me, in the same way I'm unnerved by sightings of other men I once loved, or wanted to love. Walking through a mall, or along a downtown street, I see a glimpse of hair, or a shrug, or I hear a laugh or catch a whiff of fragrance, and I get dizzy and shaky until he turns or speaks and I realize that, no, of course, it's only a stranger.

Then I'm glad, because it's easier that way.

A friend tells his story:

Climbing the stairs in the Michigan Union, he sees, descending toward him, the face and body of a woman with whom many years earlier he did more than clean chalkboards.

They spent months together, and even lived together for a glorious but contentious five days.

He has to decide, and decide quickly: Say something? Or say nothing?

He worries she won't recognize him — with bifocals now, and a white moustache, and other inevitable evidence of middle age. But more than that, he worries she'll recognize him — even call him by name — but won't remember what he remembers, in the idealized way he remembers it.

In the flash of a second, he thinks all these things.

And moves on. But he stops at the landing to turn and watch her move away from him.

Our encounters were different — mine with a boy I never knew, his with a woman he knew intimately. But he didn't regret his decision. And I don't regret mine.

Why say anything, when there's nothing to say? Why ruin memory and fantasy with words?

March 1, 1993

Love's fractured fantasy

Once again, my upstairs neighbor was slamming his girlfriend's head against the floor.

Once again, I called the cops and stepped into the hall to wait for them. Mrs. Cochrane, the genteel 70-year-old who lived across the way, was waiting, too. Dressed in a pink robe and half-glasses, she brandished a frying pan. She wanted to beat down his door and let him have it as if he were a cockroach.

Suddenly the girlfriend rushed in tears from his apartment and stumbled down the stairs, her purse and a travel bag slung over her shoulder, mascara and blood smudging her face.

"Why, dearie?" Mrs. Cochrane beseeched her as she passed us. "Why do you stay with that lout?"

The young woman looked at us with scorn, then shouted as she flung herself into the night: "Because I love him!"

You have to wonder: Where do some women learn their definitions of love? Where did Darlene Kincer learn hers?

Kincer is the 32-year-old Detroit woman who lost an arm, a leg and an unborn baby when her boyfriend dragged her behind his van, then ran over her legs — deliberately, witnesses said.

"I've got to admit it hurts me to lose my arm and leg, and I can't walk right now, but love don't come around that often," Kincer says. "I'm in love with him. Nobody's perfect."

The woman's mother thinks she's crazy. But she must have learned about love the same way the rest of us do: from our parents and other adult couples, from TV, movies, love songs, fairy tales and advertising — none of them subtle.

Now the messages are mixed, but for years they were not: Women are defined by their men and their children. Men tend to be irresponsible and inept, but a woman who knows how to endure and forgive can tame and reform the worst of them.

Most dangerous of all, floating everywhere, are these two myths: Real love lasts forever. And love conquers all.

"We've glorified love, absolute love, unconditional love, no strings attached," says Susan McGee, director of the Domestic Violence Project in Ann Arbor. "And it's women's job to sustain that, to sacrifice themselves to that ideal. Their personal worth is really secondary."

How does McGee know this? She sees hundreds of abused women. She watches movies. She listens to oldies.

And she knows the fairy tale as well as we all do: A beautiful princess kisses a frog and — lo! — a prince emerges. How the villagers cheer! The not-so-subtle message: Women, close your eyes and pucker up to a lot of ugliness. Don't give up. Buried in that animal is a man worth loving.

It's no wonder some women, broken in pieces, still talk about love. Violent men tend to romance them in between the beatings: "I can't last a day without you. You are my everything. You're the only woman that I'll ever love." The words of the songs we grew up to.

We can dismiss battered women as crazy, or we can start telling our daughters and our sisters the truth about love.

Love is patient; love is kind. But love needn't last forever, it can't survive everything, it can't fix anyone, and if standing by a man means ruining yourself, that's anything but love.

November 4, 1993

Working at a kiss

I know a man who is asking the woman he loves to kiss him at least three times a day, soulfully, for a duration of at least 20 seconds per kiss.

She is negotiating.

In my youth, we kissed or we didn't. We did not negotiate about it. If your partner wouldn't kiss you as much as you hoped, you said good-bye, no explanations necessary.

This man and the woman he loves are 30-ish. She has two children, 5 and 7. They maintain separate homes; they work more than full-time jobs. Both are busy, and they don't have much privacy. Despite that, he believes that squeezing in a full minute of serious kissing per day ought to be easy.

He also believes that even though he has to ask for it, it ought to come naturally. If it doesn't come naturally now, how will it happen at all after 10 years?

That's where we are, my husband and I — about 10 years into our partnership. I confess that on most days, we do not kiss for one full minute.

Admitting this makes me feel uneasy. My common sense tells me we're little different than other veteran couples, but my insecurity wonders if everybody doesn't kiss more than we do. What does it say that we who love each other can't muster a minute for kisses while squandering hours on activities far less satisfying?

Don't get me wrong: We mark our comings and goings with plenty of little niblet kisses that add up to maybe 15 seconds, but they're not the long involved ones the man I know would like. Those kisses require concentration. A lover who aims to please can offer a kiss while clutching clothing bound for the dry cleaners, or while wondering if the onions sauteing on the stove have turned brown, but the other will sense a distraction.

It's easy to tell a distracted kiss: It just sits there. Even an insincere kiss makes a minimal effort at exploration.

Couldn't it be argued that two people in love should be able to command each other's full attention for a 20-second kiss? Let the onions burn! Let the dry cleaning lie around another day! In the movies, lovers sweep breakfast onto the floor for the sake of a tabletop kiss. Who, I wonder, cleans up the mess? Answer: The stagehands.

If life were a stage and all the men and women on it merely players, with stagehands to do the laundry and mow the lawn and feed the children, a minute of passionate kissing might seem short.

If life were a movie, none of us would ever have morning mouth, or garlic breath, or canker sores or deadlines. In the movies, even 19th-Century cowboys kiss women long and hard: cowboys who never heard of Scope, whose teeth were rotting in their mouths, and whose breath tasted like Trigger's.

But life's no movie. On most of the days of our lives, a simple peck and a quick "Bye, honey!" seem honest and practical and adequate. After a while, I wanted to tell my naive friend, nobody counts or times kisses anymore. The measure of a marriage or any long love is taken by more complicated and less tangible markers — although, I wanted to add, there will be days when nothing is better than the surprise of one sincere singular kiss.

July 3, 1994

Hearts beat, and beat the odds

That boxer Evander Holyfield survived 12 rounds with a flawed heart is, his doctor declared, "an absolute miracle." When Holyfield announced his forced retirement Tuesday, the doctor added: "It's hard enough to fight in perfect condition."

Ha! The world is full of absolute miracles. Whose heart isn't flawed by scars, open wounds, fibrillations of devotion and desire?

A few people have it easy: They don't have to test their hearts often.

But others, startled, find themselves called upon to go much longer than 12 rounds, their hearts straining through endless matches against opponents who never tire.

In tiny Marlette, Mich., for example, Dick Sullivan still sleeps in the same room with his adult son, John, who was struck by lightning on a golf course when he was 17 and went without breath for more than 10 minutes. Dick still carries John's 6-foot-4 body across the room to the bathroom, where he sits on the edge of the tub to wash John's body and scrub his hair.

I met Dick and Marcia Sullivan about 100 days after the storm on the golf course, when doctors were warning that John would never emerge from his coma. His parents refused to concede. They sold their dairy cows and the 250-acre farm that had been in their family for generations. They built an addition on their house for John. They've earned no salary except the $4 an hour the state pays them to care for their first-born child.

Nine years later, John can't speak or walk, but smiles and responds a bit to voices. The Sullivans note his progress, and work for more. They will never institutionalize him. He is their son.

In the kitchen of an Ann Arbor sorority, a 60-year-old woman washes dishes and cleans up after the young women who live there, then goes home to take care of the 2- and 3-year-old children of a relative too strung out on drugs to care. The children are the 14th and 15th she has raised, only five of whom were her own. She sees no end in sight. She considers it her responsibility.

In Dearborn Heights, on her 40th wedding anniversary, my mother did six loads of laundry — the dirty clothes and soiled underwear of my three living grandparents, all residents of the same nursing home. For years, she and my dad cared for and visited them almost daily. Now, only one grandma remains alive, lost in muddled memories.

In courthouses and hospitals, people with beat-up and bruised hearts hope for good news but brace themselves for bad. They've been punching their way through life without notice or applause. Unlike Holyfield, they're not paid millions. Most of the time they're not even paid respect.

Quieter dramas unfold on every block in every city and town. In one corner, average people with no special training. In the opposite corner, life and all its surprise challenges: love, loss, disease, decline, responsibility. Men and women whose hearts feel achy with anxiety or loneliness keep hauling their bodies out of bed and sending them off to work, to live another day. Who can guess at their motivation?

What an absolute miracle they last so long.

April 28, 1994

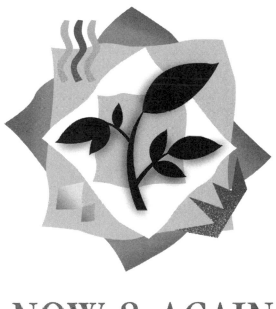

NOW & AGAIN

Wired together

Each evening, after she sings her son to sleep and kisses him good night, Kate pads downstairs in her nightgown and turns on her computer. In the purple glow of its screen, she types, finding men around the world whose words turn her on, and now, to her amazement, a man she believes is the love of her life.

His name is John, and he lives in England.

On April 11, they plan to meet: He is 45, a civil engineer, separated from his wife, father of two young boys. She is 41, the owner of a small business in suburban Detroit, never married, the single mother of an adopted handicapped 11-year-old boy.

John sent her a photo she keeps in her wallet. He's at his desk in a striped shirt and tie, certificates on the wall behind him. He's an average-looking guy, unsmiling, slightly balding.

She sent him a photo, too. Hers is from the waist up, naked, her arms lifting her long gray hair above her head. She describes herself on-line as having "voluptuous breasts with a body to match."

Since November, when they met on CompuServe's Human Sexuality Forum, John and Kate — his real name, not hers — have exchanged two or three E-mail letters each day. She types hers at night, after her son is asleep, usually two pages.

He comes to his office an hour early to read her mail and reply. Very often she gets out of bed at 3 a.m., to check for what she knows he will post by 8 a.m. British time.

She prints his letters and saves them by the month in a many-pocketed, multicolored folder now more than an inch thick.

She reads and reads and rereads them again. She can quote them from memory. She recites them in her mind. Sometimes she takes a printout into the tub, then refiles it, wrinkled from the humidity.

She has never seen John in the flesh — or in 3D, as cybernauts call it. But she is convinced he loves her deeply, and that she loves him, too.

Yet, as April 11 approaches, she feels nervous. With her son's loose-leaf paper, she made a calendar, and each day crosses off a box. "I worry," she says, "that I'm never going to be as good in bed as I am with words."

Kate came of age when many women chose adventure over security. Always busty, she attracted attention in her youth, and spent her 20s in New York City, sexually daring, willing to try anything.

Then AIDS hit, and she lost her closest friends. "A whole part of my life vanished," she wrote me on E-mail. "No one to sit with and recall memories. People I had planned to grow old with didn't make it to 35."

She vowed to be celibate. She adopted her son when he was 4 months old. She gained more than 100 pounds.

Celibacy, to Kate, did not mean self-denial. She learned how to give herself pleasure in a variety of ways. Every day, and sometimes several times over.

When she first joined CompuServe last fall, and stepped into the advanced level of the Human Sexuality Forum, she arrived with more experience and fewer inhibitions than most participants. An estimated 2,000 users check in each night, and organizers say the advanced forum has more than 87,000 members around the world.

Here's how it works: When you're in, your name appears on a list of those on-line. You may select a nickname for yourself, but not disguise your gender.

You can send a message to anyone instantly. Women are bombarded with invitations to chat, with opening lines as simple as "Hiya!" or as gushy as "Kate's the most beautiful name I've ever heard." Some are straightforwardly coarse.

Kate didn't like coarse, but she loved the rest: "It's kind of fun to have people come on to you when it's safe."

She liked to turn conversations sexual quickly, to play with words, to captivate men's attention. To seduce them. She says they seemed turned on by her direct manner.

In the beginning she juggled four conversations, each in its own corner of her screen, dumping the boring, coaxing the intriguing.

Soon she had to devise standards: No men under 33. No German men. No men from Texas. No men named Richard, her brother's name. And — she giggles — no men named Joe, a second-grade classmate "who ate paste and picked his nose."

With men she particularly liked she made dates. They would meet on-line late at night to chat, sometimes about world events, sometimes about men and women, sometimes about sex in an intellectual or clinical way. Sometimes she instructed a man how to please his wife, or encouraged another to keep trying. In the right mood, they would use words erotically, stimulating each other across thousands of miles in the flash of a second.

Kate began to savor "this time in my life when men finally seem to appreciate me for my intellect and my nature."

Kate believes computer relationships deepen far more quickly than those in real life. Nothing interferes with the words you type. Your reader can imagine whatever he wants. He is focused on you, and you on him. Because you do not look into his eyes, you feel free to say more.

Some on-line friends have come to Detroit to meet her. She has shared lunch or dinner with a handful of men, her first 3D dates in a decade, bringing her son along. No sparks ignited, no fireworks went off, but they remain friends on-line.

One man came all the way from Germany. She had warned him explicitly about her weight, nearly 300 pounds, but at the airport, she watched his face fall.

"Disappointed?" she asked.

"I guess I didn't believe you," he replied.

They spent an awkward weekend together. She was glad to see him go.

And then she met John.

For the first two weeks, they shared only sexual fantasies, alternating, his then hers, his oddly punctuated with hyphens.

Both were startled at how reliably they turned each other on with words.

After two weeks of computer sex, he wanted more. He wanted to get to know her life: "Can we have a question and answer session eventually, PLEASE?"

She has since told him everything, all the uncomfortable parts of her sexual past, why she adopted a child, why she started her business and how she struggles with it.

He has told her of his marriage — he says he was always faithful

— and of his own boys, 7 and 11, of his work and his limited sexual experience. He tells her he loves her and wants to move to Michigan, get a job and be with her.

What does she appreciate most about him? "He listens to me. I'll write him pages and pages and pages, and his one sentence tells me he read a certain long paragraph and understood what I was saying. Or he'll take pieces from letters a long time ago and pull them together."

He does what every woman wants: He pays attention.

His words roll over her like waves.

"I feel my whole being is inside you - being loved and pampered inside your body - every sensation you feel, I feel - every orgasm that flows through you, flows through me - this isn't sex, it isn't even sexy in the normal way - it's emotional fusion - tell me what you feel, Kate - I don't ever want it to stop …"

A few weeks ago, empowered by their E-mail passion, they decided to meet face-to-face. On-line users know that 3D meetings are a challenge: Nothing you've done on-line necessarily counts. You begin from scratch.

Kate planned one visit for early May, but agreed to April after he decided he couldn't wait. He'll stay 12 days for her whirlwind tour of spring in Michigan.

And she plans to have intercourse with him like she hasn't had in a decade.

She is fantasizing about it already, spending nearly 2½ hours at her keyboard daily, most of it with John, none of it seducing strangers anymore.

He tells her: "When I stagger into the arrivals area with suitcases and confused expression, just remember that inside me is that guy who writes all this stuff - you know how I think and how I love you."

And she tells him: "I have become completely confident that we will get on as well in 3D as we do here. That you will fall in love with me and I with you all over again, that you will find work here, and we will grow old together.

"I think I have spent my whole life preparing for this time … I love you in ways I find mystifying and wonderful. I love you with the giddiness of a 16-year-old girl, and the passion of a 40-year-old woman."

Her mother is terrified Kate's heart will be broken.

Kate is not so worried.

"I've always taken risks," she says, picking at a salad over lunch with me. "Curiosity is my middle name." She is trying to lose weight, and plans to get her hair cut for the first time since she was a child. She's buying new clothes, too, even lingerie for "that first night when maybe being naked will be a little more than I can handle."

In the meantime, Kate and John do their best to keep their passion up as reason works to weigh it down.

"You know there is a little part of me that's scared to death to meet you," she wrote to him a few weeks ago. Why risk what's good as it is?

Their bodies — the thousand idiosyncrasies of behavior and manner — could betray their hearts.

He wrote back. She taped his words to the countertop on which her computer sits: "I know what you mean: Sometimes I am so excited about the prospect of meeting you, but very occasionally the optimism slips and I think, 'What are you playing at, John? GROW UP!'

"It doesn't last long, though - I read one of your mails and melt, wanting to touch you, and taste you, and love you …"

March 26, 1995

Wired together, in 3D

He was the last one off the plane from London, and as she waited and waited, two fears filled her head: She had somehow failed to recognize him, and he her, and he had walked right past her. Or — worse — he had emerged far enough down the jetway to see her and, no longer interested, had turned around.

But then, there he was.

Without a word they kissed, these E-mail lovers who had never met in the flesh, in what cybernauts call 3D.

While they waited for his bags, they kissed. They kissed, it seems now, for almost 12 days straight, except when they were laughing, or trying to dig themselves out of a snowdrift, or reading aloud from books about love.

Looking back, John told a friend, "The physical touch was like placing the final piece in a jigsaw."

And Kate told me: "It was kind of like eating Kraft macaroni and cheese or wearing old shoes — warm, comfortable and familiar. It wasn't an exciting time of discovering differences, but of discovering sameness. Reassuring, familiar sameness."

I wrote about Kate and John a month ago, when they had fallen in love but hadn't met. When John planned to cross an ocean to visit her, Kate fantasized a ring, a marriage proposal on the spot, and happy ever after.

I'd like to report that happened.

But life is not a romance novel.

Things go slowly in real life. People — especially men — do not often act impulsively. Fears and insecurities must be scaled and conquered. Men and women circle each other, judge each other and test each other before they climb into the same life together.

Do not mark your calendars with a wedding date for Kate and John.

They, however, have marked the middle two weeks of this April as having been the best half-month of their lives — despite some misadventures.

They met in CompuServe's Human Sexuality Forum last fall and began an intimate, passionate and daily exchange of E-mail, writing words that stirred them, emotionally and physically.

John lives in England, works as a civil engineer and is in the throes of ending an 18-year marriage. Kate lives in suburban Detroit, runs a small business and parents an adopted boy who is mentally retarded, which is why she prefers not to use her real name here. She has never been married but is quite sexually experienced — although she swore off intercourse a decade ago, afraid of AIDS.

She also weighs nearly 300 pounds. She was terrified he would bristle at touching her. She was terrified she couldn't be as good in bed as she was with words.

But no.

He did not blink at her size, although he weighs far less. As she drove to a hotel that first night, he laid his hand on her belly.

She flinched. "I wanted him to pretend like my stomach didn't exist — to love me and just not notice that part. But he kept doing it, and I realized he touched me there because he loved me, and even that part of me."

That night, they ate grapes and chocolate kisses and cold chicken curry Kate made in advance. She put bubble bath in the hotel Jacuzzi and by the time they got to bed, they made love with ease and comfort.

On Easter morning, when they joined her family at church, her parents were wary of John. He evaded their crisp questions about his intentions. Even Kate felt a little disappointed John did not proclaim his love.

"He is British," she told herself. "He is reserved."

Kate had planned a romantic tour of all her favorite spots in northern Michigan, "but everything we wanted to do went wrong."

Their first night on the road, they missed a reservation at a fine Mission Peninsula restaurant by five minutes. And an elegant hotel where she had booked a room denied any record of it.

Later in the week in the Upper Peninsula, on a snowy dirt road leading to the Pictured Rocks National Lakeshore, John drove their rented red Mark VIII a little too wildly, and they ended up stuck.

Stuck overnight, for 20 hours.

Stuck in the snow and the cold. With some cheeses and candies and a bottle of wine and a loaf of bread. While Kate had her period. With no toilet paper but the tissue from a box of shoes Kate had bought at an outlet mall.

They slept in the backseat, wrapped in wool blankets, singing to each other, oddly unafraid. "If I die tomorrow," John whispered to Kate, "I will have died a happy man."

But as in every good movie, they were rescued, their colossal red car pulled from the snow by a tow-truck driver who couldn't stop laughing. They went on to finish their Michigan tour: Rolling through Marquette, skinny-dipping till dawn in the pool of a nearly empty UP hotel, making out in a men's store dressing room, stopping for an Elks Club fish fry in tiny Newberry, reading aloud to each other of sex and love and relationships, in bed, over dinner.

Staying up late every night. Waking up early each morning.

John did not propose, as Kate had hoped. But they dreamed out loud of a future together. He even interviewed for an engineering job in Grand Rapids after she sent his resume to scores of local firms.

They talked about buying a cabin up north. Or moving to New Zealand, with her boy and his two. He promised to build her a house grander than any they saw in Grosse Pointe. Her son called him Daddy, and he didn't mind.

He left a week ago today. She cried out all the moisture in her body, but after a good night's sleep — her first in two weeks — she found she did not ache for him. "I feel quite content and happy, secure in your love," she E-mailed him. "Your body is gone, but that's all."

He deliberately left behind his after-shave, Eau Savage. Kate sprays it on her pillow, and the keyboard of her computer.

He took with him, he says, a scant few mementos: "An Easter card. Photos, of course. A snowmobiler's glove I found when we got stuck in the snow. And strands of her hair on my clothes."

Since he left, she pesters him a little about marriage. "December 2?" she asks. He tells her to cool her jets, to have patient faith in him.

"Kate has gone into classic Female Marriage Mode," he tells me via E-mail, describing himself as "marriage-phobic," but adding "I'll get over it. Bit by bit I expect we will shuffle the practicalities and move toward being together.

"That is what I hope for."

One date is marked on their calendars: July 23. Unless cataclysmic disillusionment overcomes them, or Fate intervenes, Kate and her son leave that day for a month with John.

He tells them it's the most beautiful time of year.

April 30, 1995

Postscript: Within months, Kate and her child had moved to England. The last I heard from her on E-mail, she and John were building a home by the sea and talking, still tentatively, about marriage.

Giftless Christmas

Not one of the economic forecasters called upon to predict the size of Christmas spending this year has noticed my family's new approach: No gifts at all.

Sometimes I suspect we are on the bold cutting edge of a trend that will stun retailers who seem to think the more money you have, the more you'll spend on gaudy jewelry, cashmere sweaters, espresso machines and Salad Shooters. Won't those merchants howl when they realize how many of us don't need or want yet more stuff in our lives?

But sometimes I think my family is just … dysfunctional.

Does our No-Gift Christmas mean we are more secure in each other's affection than the average family? Or does it suggest we're self-centered, too absorbed in our own petty lives to plan or shop? The worst possibility is that it means we just don't care like we used to.

"That's it!" my husband said wryly as I wrung my hands over our new plan, which my mother suggested sometime in July. "You should have tackled your mother and shouted, 'No! No! We want to buy more for each other this Christmas because we love each other so much more than we did last year!'

"But you didn't do that because you obviously don't love each other anymore. So now that the truth is out, why not save your money?"

The truth is, we're not really out to save money, although that will be nice, especially for my brother and his wife, whose gift to each other will be a new dishwasher, theirs having died in May.

Mostly we're out to save anxiety and guilt and a sense of "enough, already!" My mother said she decided to proclaim a No-Gift Christmas when, having entered her 60s, she looked around her home and saw too many miniature pewter figurines, too many special-occasion serving dishes, fancy bread boards, driving gloves, etc., etc.

She didn't want anything else. And my dad has never wanted anything except the love of his children, his daily newspaper and a Snickers before bed.

We've tried other Christmases:

■ The $10 Christmas. None of us remembers what we gave or got, although my mother insists she was the only one who followed the rule.

■ The Make-It-Yourself Christmas, which also allowed the giving of previously owned things. I think I'm the only one who complied, giving my sister-in-law one of my extra cookie sheets, and slaving over a hot stove to make mustards and jams nobody liked.

The No-Gift Christmas is yet another experiment, limited to adults only. We'll continue to buy toys for the boys, my nephews Christopher and Brian, who at 6 and 7 still believe more is better because they've never had to stage a garage sale.

So far this year everyone in my family — including me when I shut off the second-guessing — reports an unusual euphoria. Part of it is relief from all those enduring Christmas questions: Is this good enough? Didn't I get him one like that four years ago? Will they think me cheap? Or weird?

Mostly, though, it's knowing we're creating our own Christmas, unbullied by profiteers, unswayed by sentimental Christmas advertising. On Christmas morning at my brother's place in Minnesota, where normally we take turns unwrapping things, all we'll have to open is our hearts.

November 30, 1993

Giftless Christmas: How it went

Only 355 planning days left till next Christmas. And it's never too early to make dramatic changes in how you celebrate, and how you feel later.

One friend described her Christmas: "It was just too much. It's like an orgy: You feel good while it's happening, but afterward you feel sick."

In my family, we avoided most post-Christmas malaise by happily staging our First Annual Giftless Christmas.

Cynics predicted someone would cheat, making the rest of us feel like cheap fools. Or we'd feel so bereft that we'd spend twice as much at post-Christmas sales.

Wrong.

Oh, there were gifts, I guess you'd call them. In mid-December my mother gave each of us a hefty jar of homemade chocolate-caramel ice cream topping. And, a studio portrait of her and Dad wrapped in a manila envelope. She insisted neither was a Christmas gift.

My brothers exchanged identical Sierra Club desk calendars, as they have for 15 years, since they were once embarrassed to have bought each other the same thing. Now it's a tradition, immutable.

We did not feel bored or deprived as we watched the boys, 6 and 7, tear open dozens of packages, though we concluded maybe their Christmas was too bountiful. My dad remarked as wrapping paper flew: "I remember when I got only an orange for Christmas."

We harbored no guilt over gifts that weren't right. We spent more time talking, retelling stories, revealing secret dreams. My brother and I took a long walk in 10-below-zero cold.

That night, my mother announced time for "the grab bag." She had foraged her home for enough little things — most unused — to wrap three gifts for each of us, which we selected from a basket she carried around the room. On first round, my 7-year-old nephew got Gillette shaving cream. I got a man's deodorant stick. My brother got a spray bottle of White Shoulders, my grandma's favorite, found unopened in her nightstand after she died.

For 10 minutes we laughed and bartered our gifts if we could. My husband traded his Oil of Olay for a year-old fruitcake. Everyone ended up with something they could use — or save for subsequent grab bags.

This was a technical violation. But Mom didn't care who got what, or whether they liked it. She spent no money or anxiety on her grab bag.

Our giftlessness liberated us. I surprised myself two evenings by driving around just to look at lights. I wrote better notes to distant friends. I hummed while I baked. I felt zero panic and more joy.

For the first time, my husband and I exchanged no gifts, either. I felt stricken when friends seemed shocked. But I realized it meant nothing more than no compulsion to prove our love.

Watching a short video of our holiday, we were struck by how much of it focused on food: Amazing shrinking coffee cakes. Trays of cookies decimated by day's end, refreshed by Mom by morning. Steaming platters of pierogi, kielbasa, chicken wings, salmon.

On Christmas Day afternoon, shoving yet another wedge of cheese into his mouth, my brother had a bright idea: "Next year, how about a foodless Christmas!"

Soon, we'll have this thing tamed.

January 4, 1994

The mystery of Juan's pencil

Who is Juan Lelito? And why is his pencil on my kitchen counter? On one of its six edges is Juan's name, carved in tiny pinpricks, as if Juan were a bored schoolkid. Or a factory worker with nothing better to do over lunch.

But how did his pencil get to my house?

Actually, all the pencils in our house sneaked in. Neither my husband nor I remembers buying a single pencil in our 10 years together, yet a couple of dozen clutter our desks and our kitchen.

No wonder Mom always told me not to chew on my pencil: Think of the hands that hold it over its lifetime, each user paying it equal disregard.

A pencil Isiah Thomas used to jot down a friend's phone number might be one a kid finds on the street to work multiplication problems. The pencil with which Rush Limbaugh scrawls middle-of-the-night insights may end up in Hillary Clinton's hand, working a crossword puzzle.

Nobody feels possessive about pencils. Who wonders, as they check out of a motel, "Did I pack my pencil?"

But Juan, he wanted that pencil to be his. That's why he put his name on it.

Curious, I look in the phone book. No Lelito.

Then I call the company that manufactured the pencil, figuring that's what Columbo would do.

Dixon Ticonderoga produces 288 million pencils a year at its plant in the Ozarks. A Dixon Ticonderoga is considered the Cadillac of pencils, an amiable woman named Laura Van Camp tells me: more expensive than other pencils, distinctive because of its patented ferrule.

Its what? The ferrule is the ridged band of metal where the eraser meets the wood; Dixon Ticonderoga makes theirs bright green and yellow. That, she says, makes the pencil popular with Hollywood producers.

"One of our favorite pastimes here is watching TV shows and

movies to see how many Ticonderogas we can spot," she says. "Now you'll start doing it! You'll watch 'Murphy Brown' and see those Ticonderogas on her desk."

Aha! I think. Perhaps Juan is a cameraman for "Murphy Brown."

But then I talk to someone else at the company who tells me Juan's pencil is unusual because it is a No. 3, extra hard. Those constitute only 1½ percent of Dixon Ticonderoga's production, and are preferred by engineers and draftsmen, especially in California.

Aha! I think. Perhaps Juan is an out-of-work aerospace engineer, secretly seeing Candice Bergen. When her husband finds Juan's pencil on their kitchen counter, he throws it out the window. A vacationing retired insurance claims adjuster, touring the neighborhoods of the rich and famous, spots the pencil on the street and pockets it as a souvenir. Back in Detroit, though, he inadvertently leaves it on a Midas Muffler counter, where I pick it up and carry it home.

Implausible, yes. Impossible, no.

My imagination works on Juan's pencil for several days. I bring it to the office. I show it around. I keep my friends up to date on my theories until, suddenly, one day I look for it and it is gone.

Not in my pencil jar. Not in my drawer. Not in my purse.

Juan's pencil is on the loose again. Pick it up if you see it, will you?

October 4, 1994

Juan Lelito, found

Turns out everybody knows Juan Lelito but me.

I heard from ex-girlfriends, coworkers, wives of business associates and high school chums after I wrote last week about finding a pencil carved with his name on my kitchen counter. Most of those who know Juan described him as "unusual," although one woman called him "weird."

I had speculated that Juan was a bored schoolkid or a bored factory worker. When manufacturers of the Dixon Ticonderoga pencil told me it was popular with Hollywood producers, and often appeared on Murphy Brown's desk, I wondered if Juan was a cameraman. Then I learned the No. 3 pencil is popular with engineers and draftsmen, and figured Juan was an out-of-work aerospace engineer who … well, anyway, I concocted elaborate fantasies about Juan.

My first call on the day the column ran announced, "You found me!"

Juan Lelito is chief engineer for the Detroit-Windsor tunnel, hired 3½ years ago to orchestrate the 64-year-old tunnel's $30-million renovation. He's 44, divorced and a man about town, although his phone number is unlisted, which is why I couldn't find him in local phone directories.

He attends many meetings, which last many minutes. To pass the time, he pokes holes in his pencils with the tip of a pen, specifically a Berol Extra-Fine pen. "No other pen works," he insists. Eventually the holes spell his name. He guesses he has carved at least 20 pencils with his name in the last few years.

He has carved his name, too, on picnic tables and on trees in hunting blinds, "whenever I'm bored," with a tiny inch-and-a-half pocket knife he keeps on his key ring.

"It's a nice-sounding name," says Juan. His father carried mixed Polish and Italian blood, with a dab of Spanish, and took on "Juan" as a middle name during World War II. Then he passed it to his son, who says, "I would have to do a few months in therapy to figure out why I carve it so much."

As for how his pencil got to my house, two theories emerged as we talked:

■ Last spring he helped a friend install software on her home computer. She happens to be a freelance writer for the Free Press business section, which is down the hall from my office.

■ About the same time, he dated a woman who lives in the same town I do, dined with her in some of the same restaurants where I eat, and once left his van for a brake job at a local Midas Muffler. Because he carries his pencils in his pants pockets — which struck me as a little weird — "they sometimes fall out," he said.

However I acquired Juan's Lelito's pencil, I didn't have it for long. It vanished before I wrote the column about it, and that's the saddest part of Juan's story: All the pencils on which he has carved his name have vanished, off into that never-never land of junk drawers, pencil jars, linty purse bottoms, the dark dusty spaces between desks and walls. He hasn't been able to hang onto a single one.

A therapist would certainly have something to say about that.

October 11, 1994

A month in the country

Nobody needs a month away less than I do.

My work is neither back-breaking, heart-wrenching nor nerve-wracking.

At home I tend no needy dependents, neither children, nor aging parents, nor a slugabed husband.

I'm no Superwoman. I'm not exhausted. And I'm not at my wit's end.

But I'm taking a month off, starting today, and I feel truly blessed.

I work for a company that lets me take the time on top of my paid vacation. And the financial health of my household is sturdy enough to indulge this.

It's a tradeoff: time instead of money. For me, it's a chance to remember who I am apart from my work, to take off the costume of Susan Ager, columnist, and investigate what else hangs in my closet.

In the early '70s, as I was entering the work world, I heard a line that went something like this: "You can be a worker, or you can be a lover, but it's hard to be both." I had a suspicion what it meant, but now I know for sure.

Even work you love tends to suck away your prime hours. You're left with scraps from which to muster love for your family, your friends, the larger world around you. My husband and I sometimes joke that we get the worn-out, beaten-down, squeezed-dry husks of each other, the parts left over from work. We who love each other best deserve better than dregs.

I'm inspired by stories about people who redefine success, who drop out and slow down. A couple of years ago I read a classic book called "Living the Good Life," by Scott and Helen Nearing, who abandoned New York City for a maple sugar farm in New Hampshire, then built their own stone home and barns in Maine.

In that book were these words: "Money must be paid for, just like everything else."

I think about my money, and what it costs. I make money, but my friends often feel abandoned. I write columns, but I lack the energy and will to write letters, or sometimes even to buy a birthday card on time. I create sentences, but no art or music or anything that will last. I measure my life by achievement at work and let the most vital relationships of my life languish.

I cry and shout too often over nonsense.

A month away will hardly fix all that. It won't be "A Year in Provence," and hardly worth a book, let alone a column or two. But it will remind me of who else I am besides a worker.

I'll spend the month at our little cottage, just 330 square feet. I love it because in it only essentials fit. It has no TV, no microwave, no clock. Trash must be carried up our 62 steps, so we're careful about what we carry down.

My husband will spend half the days with me. But I look forward to being alone, too. I'll try to walk a few miles every day, for a change. I'll write letters and hope for letters back. I'll read more, and think more vigorously, I hope, because my thinking muscles feel flabby lately.

I'll reacquaint myself with the stars, the black snake that lives on our rocks, and the ducks that nibble my toes. Maybe I'll name a few more trees and wildflowers. Maybe, when the grapes ripen in mid-September, I'll make pies.

I plead guilty to small goals. For 30 days I will be happy to wake up in the morning, without plans, and simply live.

I'm blessed, I know. I wish everyone could do this. And I wonder why those who could don't.

August 22, 1993

Lessons from the country

Sometimes we have to slow down to learn the simplest lessons. I've been away for a month, living most of the time alone in a tiny cottage on a big lake, 20 minutes from the nearest newspaper or Big Mac, without TV or movies or deadlines or obligations.

The most dramatic moments of the month were these:

At the local supermarket, I watched a Mennonite man and his adolescent son, both in long pants, suspenders and hats, unload from their shopping cart 45 loaves of soft, white bread. The bread was on sale, three for a dollar, and they bought nothing else.

One dusk, I watched a great blue heron, four feet tall, walk to the end of our dock, dive down and come up with a fish in its beak as big as my hand. It flipped the fish into its mouth, and I watched that shape lurch down its long throat until the heron bent over for a few sips of lake water and a tremendous swallow that forced the fish into its belly.

I finished my own dinner more slowly.

What else did I learn in a month?

■ Loneliness is like the wind. It sneaks up on you, at times in ferocious gusts, but if you wait, calm returns.

■ Nothing beats loneliness like baking. Failure is rare, and you end up with something you can give away.

■ You can provide good company by talking to yourself. I don't understand how it got such a bad reputation. It feels good, and is no more crazy than masturbation.

■ Clean windows make a difference, especially if the sun pours through them in the morning. I put off washing ours because the job involves hauling a stepladder around and confronting spiders and wasps. But one day I did them, and the next morning I felt happy.

■ There is no finer supper than sweet corn, sliced tomatoes and new potatoes boiled in their skins, mashed with a fork and topped with butter and chives.

■ Life is too short to own a refrigerator that needs defrosting.

■ At 40, a woman who goes a month without a bra suffers no noticeable new droop.

■ One may live without the news, but not without the weather forecast.

■ Not too many days can pass in sheer leisure before you get the itch to achieve. Something more than writing letters or reading books. So I rescued from the side of the road an old metal lawn chair with a FREE sign on it. Once green, it had been repainted red, white, then pink. I scraped, sanded and epoxied it, then painted it royal blue.

I painted the shed door green. I planted black-eyed susans and rose of Sharon saplings. I raked and yanked poison ivy vines. Funny: The more I did, the better I felt.

■ The dirtier you get during the day, the better you sleep at night.

Since I've been home, I've tried to use what I learned, but I know it will be hard. My first day back, as I stood in the kitchen reading aloud to myself a letter a friend sent us, my husband interrupted to say, "I've read it already." I replied, "Please humor me."

Yesterday I drove to work and for the first time in my life found myself in the slow lane. I did not want to go as fast as the fast lane required. I dawdled, thinking about white bread and blue herons and sweet corn, but my horse found the way, so here I am again.

September 21, 1993

The disgusting side of puppy love

The Massachusetts guy whose dog turned up this week after fleeing a jet at Metro Airport 12 days earlier was gushy with gratitude toward everybody who helped search.

"I love Detroit now," he said, failing to explain how he felt about it earlier. "People here are special … Apparently they're all dog-lovers."

Wrong.

I would be a dog-lover if dogs knew their place and kept their tongues to themselves.

But no. Even a dog you just met wants to slobber all over your face.

Dog owners find this charming, smiling as their pup's tongue explores your facial geography. Would they be so charmed if you let your 3-year-old child lick them?

But 3-year-olds usually keep their tongues in their mouths. Dogs don't. We all know where dog tongues have been.

Dogs root around in the backyard, attracted to various droppings. They like street gutters and dark corners and places where you and I would not put our hands. They're intrigued by dead animals — mice and birds and such. And they're fascinated by what you and I would call private parts — their own and those of other dogs.

I guess dog lovers are willing to forget all this, or forgive it. They encourage their dogs to lick them. Did you see that big photo of Jeff Shotland reunited with his lost dog? Did you see how Emi was leaping up on Shotland and aiming, with her tongue, for his nose?

Or maybe it was his lips.

This, to me, is the worst: Dog lovers kiss their dogs on the lips.

I've seen it time and again. Smooch smooch smooch, oh you cute little baby, gimme a smoochie.

Life is too short for hard-and-fast rules, but this is one I live by:

Lips that touch dog lips will never touch mine.

One other thing: Dogs figure they have a right to join you in bed.

Don't let a friend with a dog spend the night unless you are ready to be startled awake by a pooch panting and scrambling to climb onto — and under — your comforter.

My stepdaughter's black Lab, Rosie, is a sweet creature, but seems surprised when we don't want to snuggle with her at 6 a.m. on Saturday. We're still asleep, but she has just finished her morning constitutional and bounds up the stairs — failing once again to wipe her feet at the door.

Too many dog lovers encourage this bed stuff. They let their pups sleep with them. They enjoy dog hair on their sheets and dog breath on their pillows.

One single woman I know lets her dog lick her ice cream cone, and sometimes shares a beer with her dog: "She licks from the bottle, and I drink after her."

Yuk.

I know, I know. I've heard the contention that human mouths contain more germs than dog mouths. I just don't believe it. If dogs brushed their teeth and gargled with Scope as often as people do, and learned to wipe their feet, and kept their noses out of nasty places, and tucked their tongues away where they belong — maybe I'd allow a little kiss now and again.

If any dog would have me.

May 9, 1996

Puppy love: In the doghouse

The dog-lovers of Michigan rose up snarling and took a chunk out of my hide for admitting in print that I don't like slobbery dogs.

Angry readers called me a cold-hearted bitch. Angrier readers called me an ugly, cold-hearted bitch, and told me to rot in hell. The angriest readers called me uglier than the ugliest dog they've ever seen, and vowed to never read my column again.

These readers — hundreds of them — were brutal to me, a stranger. But hey, they love their dogs.

What provoked this?

I wrote in my May 9 column that I know where dog tongues have been, and, therefore, don't like those tongues on my face. And I made a little fun of people who smooch their dogs on the lips. The headline — which I didn't write — used the word "disgusting." But I only used the word "yuk." And only once.

My column appeared the day after the Free Press ran a Page One spread on a dog named Emi, found after 12 days roaming near Metro

Airport. It included a huge photo of Emi leaping up to lick her owner's face.

Some readers contended I ruined the sweet story for them. "You wiped the smile right off my face," one woman hissed.

Geez. I'm sorry. Don't get me wrong: I'm glad the guy got his dog back. I'm happy for anyone who has a dog to love. Contrary to suggestions from some readers, I have owned dogs, including a poodle who followed me home from school and became part of the family, and have good memories of others, including a 16-year-old beagle who liked to nap in my lap.

I've even mailed sympathy cards to friends whose beloved pets have died.

But I don't want a dog's tongue on my face, OK?

Some readers agreed, including several who train their dogs to mind their place. That means no jumping on people, no licking them, no sniffing their crotches. These dog-lovers suggested the problem is not dogs but their indulgent owners.

A few other dog-owners laughed over the column, including one woman who said: "My dog is partial to my husband's toes, and while I love my husband, I don't want to lick his toes, nor do I want to kiss my dog after my dog has licked his toes."

I expected disagreement about dog tongues, but I didn't expect people who love pooches to be so nasty to a human being like me.

Said one woman: "We knew you were a little strange when you refused to wear any makeup to improve your appearance, but now we know you're as ugly on the inside as the outside."

Another: "No animal or human being could ever love you."

Another: "All a dog would have to do is take one good look at your face and he'd throw up all over you."

One guy got on the phone with his dog, Einstein, and egged him on: "Bark at the mean lady! Bark at her!" Einstein complied.

I decided not to take any of this personally.

But while I make light of it here, it troubles and mystifies me.

Where does this meanness come from? Do these people talk like this to those they love who happen to disagree with them? Or is this about something deeper and more sinister?

I sense in society a free-wheeling rage, a boiling anger at nothing in particular but everything in general.

It swells in people. It throbs. And then my words, or anybody's words, press up against the fury like a finger pressing hard on a boil.

And because it has nowhere else to go, it erupts.

May 21, 1996

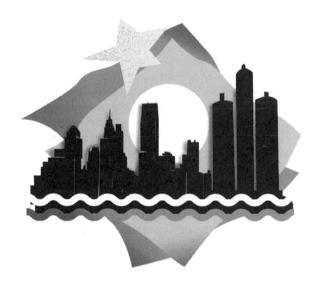

THE MOTOR CITY

Quitters sometimes win

For a long time I considered Coleman Young a sad and foolish man for failing to recognize that his prime had passed.

The City of Detroit is ailing physically and spiritually. But Young, turning 75 today, lacks the fire to turn much around anymore.

To run again for mayor, he risks humiliation. Polls show almost 80 percent of Detroit voters think he should retire.

But lately I've realized, hell, we're all the same. None of us ready to admit we're past our prime. Few of us able to quit at the right time.

I talk with a friend whose marriage has gasped for life so long it's turning blue. Yet the marriage continues, my friend unable to retire it.

I know others whose relationships are, by their own account, superficial, unsatisfying or even dangerous — but who can't or won't quit. They tell themselves there's hope. They wait for a second wind.

We all know women who used to look good in leggings, and think they still do. We all know men beyond their prime for chatting up young things, who still try.

We know bosses whose hearts have found homes in something other than their work, who ought to move over and make way for those eager to steer the ship.

Nearly everyone quits too late, after the line on the graph peaks, then begins to dip. Batting averages decline. New songs struggle but can't make it up the charts. Words don't stir readers as they used to. Half-baked decisions limp along down the line.

When they do quit, the world acts sad and disappointed for a moment. But then the whispers begin: "Whew! About time."

How terrific it would feel to quit too soon! To hear the world gasp, "No way! What a tragedy! What will we do without you?"

It's hard to think of many who've quit too soon.

Boxer Rocky Marciano, who retired undefeated, 49 and 0. Greta Garbo, who decided while still gorgeous to age in hiding. Writer J.D. Salinger, who produced a classic in "The Catcher in the Rye," wrote a few other things, then shut himself away in a home overlooking the Connecticut River.

Yet we hardly trust people like that. We wait for them to re-emerge: Surely Salinger will publish something soon.

Or we dismiss them as fearful and insecure.

I recall a story told me by a man who loved a woman who refused to discuss her age but who fretted constantly about aging. Her body was trim and nearly wrinkleless, and he guessed her to be in her mid-40s, perhaps.

One day he found her dead in her bathtub. Her driver's license revealed her to be 65.

Her note said she wanted to die while she still looked good.

I felt terribly sad for her.

Many others quit too soon, ending their lives and shocking the rest of us who were eager for more from them. Sylvia Plath, Vincent van Gogh, Marilyn Monroe, Ernest Hemingway, Abbie Hoffman, Sarah Goddard Power.

But who am I to say what's too soon? Only the human being who carries the cup can remember what used to be inside, can know what has evaporated away and can measure what's left to spend.

Alas, some of us hardly care. We hear applause. Fainter than before. But what noise remains keeps us on the stage, even though we've worn out our role, and forgotten many of our lines.

It would be reassuring to have friends who told us the truth, for our own sake. Who told us when it's time to put away the leggings. Or time to retire, if we hope to save any shred of self-respect.

But few of us can be such frank friends.

And most of us don't have them.

May 24, 1993

New mayor's victory dance

To my resolution list for 1994 I've added a fantasy: I'd like to dance with Dennis Archer, Detroit's new mayor. One dance. I'm not greedy.

I know so many men who can't dance, or who can but won't, or who could but won't let themselves. I guess they have something to fear. "No sober man dances, unless he happens to be mad," Cicero said 2,000 years ago, and by mad the wise man meant crazy.

To dance is to abandon control. To let your body do what it itches to do. To those not dancing, the dancing man looks geeky, feet in the air, elbows cocked, strutting like a chicken, or twirling till he's dizzy. But the dancing man is not distracting himself with thoughts of England or baseball or anything but the way the music makes him feel.

Dennis Archer — drunk with adrenaline — danced the other night in front of thousands. Early in the evening, he delivered on a campaign promise by granting the first dance to 76-year-old Iona Echols. She shimmied in a shimmery blue dress. Dennis shimmied back in a tux. Together they sizzled, and those watching howled at the heat.

Later, at the Inaugural Ball, Dennis took to the floor with his wife. Theirs was not the restrained one-two-one-two the Clintons did on inaugural night a year ago, when you could almost hear the First Couple counting to themselves.

The Archers danced effortlessly, exuberantly, even kissing at one turn. They danced as couples do who have spent a lifetime learning each other's rhythms. When a TV reporter asked if they had practiced for that dance, Dennis scoffed. "Are you kidding? It's like riding bicycles."

Any man who says dancing is like riding a bicycle is at ease with himself, unafraid to move, unafraid to walk down the hall near his office, to use the employee bathroom.

We might expect such a man, as mayor, to be nimble, in wit and in deed. Perhaps on spring afternoons he will bicycle through the streets of the city and scoop its residents into his arms for a turn on the pavement.

On the same day he danced, this new guy also shouted and cried. He very deliberately wiped his damp glasses after his 24-year-old son's introduction and said, before he began his own speech, "We have somewhat of a sensitive family." Not an apology, or a joke. Just a fact.

His wife was just then tucking away her wet Kleenex.

Can anyone claim these were calculated moves? Skeptics have derided Bill Clinton's tears as wet but insincere. I think they're wrong. No man cries for points, but the man who lets himself cry wins them.

We make these judgments because we hardly know Dennis Archer. We're still seeking clues to his character. So you watch a man dance, you see him wipe his eyes, you notice the way he massages his son's shoulder as the young man stands smitten with tears at a podium, and what conclusion can you draw but that you will root for him as if he were your own father or son, even if he makes mistakes?

These images last and inspire faith. They are more potent than most of a man's million words, wispy as smoke.

Detroit's dancing days are over, the cynics like to say, but even they were hushed by Dennis Archer's footwork.

So was I.

January 6, 1994

Familiar face shown the door

Since I stood in line at 16 for my first driver's license, no face has smiled down at me but Richard Austin's.

I thought Austin was forever. Like the pope, he had his job for life — and he deserved it.

But the other day, Michiganders put Richard Austin, age 81, out to pasture. While other election results upset me, this one broke my heart.

"For the first time in 24 years, Richard Austin is not at work," his longtime aide Liz Boyd told me Wednesday. "He stayed home today."

Both she and I know that for 38 years, he has lived in the same house on Oakman Boulevard in Detroit. For 55 years he has been married to the same wife, Ida. And for his 24 years as secretary of state he never took a vacation. Once he told me, "The travel between Detroit and Lansing is quite enough of a diversion."

I admit I never gave much thought to what kind of job he was doing. My renewal notices always came on time. When I had to visit a branch office, I always waited longer than I wanted to, but not as long as I feared I might. Hell, I've waited longer at doctors' offices.

Never did I hear anyone curse Richard Austin's policies or character, or blame him for the quality of their lives.

He has been displaced, I guess, because he's older and slower. In his debate with opponent Candice Miller, he rambled, confused pro-life and pro-choice and had to ask the moderator to repeat a question.

His gentlemanly personality won him no points in the campaign. Miller, who is half his age, disgraced herself at a roast by calling him "Little Dicky" and remarking that Austin had "gold in his teeth, silver in his hair and lead in his ass."

He was hurt by allegations that he failed to vote in the 1992 presidential election, a story newspapers played big, even though a day later they were proven wrong. Am I the only one who didn't care if Austin did miss an election or two? Don't we all? Is there any real relationship between voting and patriotism or goodness or competence?

Mostly I will miss Richard Austin's face because I've liked him. I interviewed him twice, once during his unsuccessful bid for the U.S. Senate in 1976, and once when he turned 75 in 1988. During that interview, I asked less about politics, and more about life.

About his old-fashioned marriage he joked, "You'd think a guy who had been secretary of state for 17 years by now would be entitled to some rights, but I still have to take out the garbage."

He told me that to stay young, "I try to have friends." And he does 15 minutes of calisthenics each day, taking time on weekends to walk eight to 10 miles on the streets of Detroit.

"My highest aspiration was to render public service," he said. The son of a coal miner, a former shoe-shine boy, Austin was proud that while as a CPA he had just 400 clients, as secretary of state he had 9 million.

When I asked if he would run again, he said sure. His health was good. His agenda was unfinished. "You'll have to tell me whether or not I'm useful."

I guess we've told him. Now they'll take down his picture and put up one of a woman I hope can grow into grace.

Maybe now Richard Austin will take a vacation. But that's probably the last thing he wants to do with his life.

November 10, 1994

A coach's worst call

Has a drunken stranger ever blown his foul breath down your neck while saying he loves you?

Have you ever stepped from the rest room of a fine restaurant as a drunk rushing in throws up on your shoes?

Have you tried to celebrate some happy event over dinner while jerks at the next table made such a ruckus you finally left in despair and rage?

I have, and people I know have, and to us Gary Moeller's behavior at a Southfield restaurant the other night was no small thing.

We wanted an apology from the U-M football coach. We wanted him to stand up, as soon as he was able. To call a press conference, gathering onto a big stage every waitress, every restaurant patron, every cop and doctor and nurse he insulted and offended and hurt. In front: his wife and children.

We wanted to hear him issue a straight, unembellished, unambiguous apology.

Anyone could have written his script:

"I want to apologize to each of you, to look in your eyes and tell you how very sorry I am that I behaved like an idiot and demeaned you as you tried to do your job or eat a quiet meal. You, on whose faith and devotion I depend for my team's livelihood and my own.

"I have no excuse for myself. I was wrong and stupid.

"And to you whom I love most — my wife, my kids — I owe the biggest apology. Please, please, forgive me."

Some have said that if everyone were punished for behavior like Moeller's, America's workplaces would empty. That's ridiculous. Most Americans over the age of 22 never get drunk. Most people stop themselves when they see trouble starting. Most people do not call their wives vulgar names in public, or dare to lay a finger on an officer of the law. Most people do not let their wives sit alone in the car for an hour while they continue to make fools of themselves inside.

This is not average behavior. Even if it were, Moeller isn't just anybody and he knows it.

I'm just a small-time columnist and people recognize me buying bras and buying bananas. I do not dare stage even the pettiest of public spats with my husband. In others' minds, and my own, I represent my employer.

I don't care what Moeller calls his wife in the privacy of their home or how much he drinks there.

But in public he carries on his chest the maize-and-blue of the University of Michigan. Could U-M President Jim Duderstadt resume his job the next day if he behaved as Moeller did? Do any of us want to work for a boss who would act like that and then, worse, wouldn't summon the guts to apologize?

A statement read by somebody else six days late is not enough. "I am deeply embarrassed" is not the same as "I am deeply sorry." The statement also said his behavior "is in no way indicative of an alcohol problem" or "any family difficulties." Amazing. If you ruin your good name in one night, isn't that a problem?

This was not one false move, but a man exploding as if a bomb went off in his belly. The fallout landed everywhere.

Let his recovery begin, in blessed privacy, beyond our eyes.

And let it begin for his family, and everyone else who had the misfortune that night to cross his sorry path.

May 7, 1995

Postscript: Moeller resigned under pressure, pleaded no contest to a charge of disorderly conduct and paid a fine. He never publicly apologized.

Sounds of engines fill the land

Amid the cheering and hoopla celebrating 100 years of automobiles in American life, may I quietly add one more thing?

The automobile has ruined the sounds of the night.

During the day, we often are too busy to notice the noise. But in the evening, when we lie on our beds, wide awake sometimes with trembling and ache, what we hear is not the shrill chirp of crickets, or the steady drip of rain. Those comforting sounds, as old as the earth, are diluted or drowned by the roar of machines man has made.

Stop and listen now, wherever you are. Chances are you will hear, behind everything else, the steady drone of tires and engines and speed. Chances are you will hear not one car or a dozen but 100 or more within your earshot.

Highways that carried 5,000 vehicles each day in the 1950s now carry 70,000. People who bought homes along those highways closed their windows at some point years ago, never to open them again. They mask traffic noise with the noise of music or TV or air conditioners.

Who sleeps with their windows wide open to the mysterious sounds of the night anymore?

Meanwhile, governments are building noise barriers, mostly along America's newest highways, at a cost of $1 million per mile. The best, built of cinder block, steel, or pre-cast concrete, muffle the noise only by half.

How soon will traffic on those roads double?

I remember clearly those few nights in my life when I fell asleep without the discomforting lullaby of traffic.

Once, years ago, I camped at Big Sur on the Pacific Ocean, in mid-winter, under the stars, far from a road. The stillness scared me.

In Peru, I slept one night at a tiny hotel in the Andes, perched on the edge of the Machu Picchu ruins. A bus deposited tourists there, then took most of them away by dusk. It did not return until morning, announcing itself for 20 minutes as it chugged up the mountainside.

I slept at a primitive lodge along the Amazon, accessible only by riverboat. I slept in a sagging old cabin on an isolated lake in Canada.

And a few weeks ago, I slept in a bed-and-breakfast on Mackinac Island. There, at the turn of the century, town fathers banned all motor vehicles.

I stayed in a third-floor room with high ceilings and a small window, and that night it rained. I lay with my eyes closed and heard rain as I've never heard it before.

I listened to it fall on the roof shingles beyond my window. I listened to it fall on the lawn below. And I swore I could hear it falling, too, in the distance, on the vast lakes that surrounded us.

The automobile has produced noisy offspring: jet engines in the sky, Jet Skis on our water, snowmobiles in our wilderness. Engines of all kinds grate on us: lawn mowers and leaf blowers and air conditioners.

Music, wires in a box, now goes wherever the automobile goes. Some suburbs try to pass laws to force kids to keep their radios down, but no law will ever quiet the automobile itself.

There's no turning back. There's only escape.

Some of us do run far, far away — driving to get there. We construct a private gravel road, and build our house on a mountainside, or on the flatlands of an empty state like Montana. Then we pray that no politician or developer bent on progress or profit ever finds our spot and builds a public road to it.

Because if you put down pavement, automobiles will find it, then fill it, and steal again the peace we used to know.

June 27, 1996

Failing, despite really trying

Whether Bill Bonds deserves my sympathy, he compels my attention. Because he belongs to us, we can watch as he fails to fix himself.

The rest of us fail privately. Thank God we can stroll through malls anonymously, hiding our bad habits, our illnesses and our screwed-up personalities under our clothes.

But when you look around you at the mall, it helps to remember that almost everybody you see is fighting — and losing — some struggle within.

"Hey, I'm human," the newscaster told reporters after his arrest Sunday on suspicion of drunk driving. "What about you guys?"

I confess. And feel grateful that my own flaws and the flaws of my friends are easier to hide or disguise. Nobody clocks our moves or counts our flubs.

Some people say Bonds deserves not a peanut of sympathy because he's always been a jerk and always will be one. My guess is that, like everyone else, he is a complicated stew of traits, except he's got one bad potato that keeps bobbing to the top of his pot.

He is captivating because he's an exquisitely flamboyant failure at self-improvement. He helps put our own quiet chronic failures in perspective.

Of course we say we want success stories. Hollywood producers have learned that test audiences will boo unhappy endings. So in movies, as in fairy tales, losers almost always win. Love prevails.

The next morning on the way to work, we make vows: To contain our temper. To smile, not snap, at the kids. No ice cream tonight. No ice cream ever! No wallowing, no staring at the ceiling. Action! Just do it!

Some people are lucky: Their bad habits have names. Alcohol. Gambling. Infidelity. Fear of failure. When a bad habit has a name, you can buy books about beating it.

Other people are plagued by things that can't be captured in a word or anecdote but keep them awake at night, wondering why they cannot get a grip.

Those are the men and women I find most interesting. Neither complacent nor smug about who they are, they take themselves on.

I like the inspiration of success stories, but I also like company.

The entire drama of human existence amounts to a struggle to live better. To find more peace within our own skins. To do more good outside ourselves. To discover the fullness of life, and face it head on, rather than hiding.

All the resolutions of our days ... if we each abided by half of them, the world would be a fabulous place. No one would take cuts, smack a child or drive drunk.

So I watch Bill Bonds and read about his latest setback with a lump of self-recognition in my throat. He's still fighting a big one, or maybe he's given up. How humiliated he must be. How angry and disappointed must be those who love him. A man with money and support from his employer and his fans still doesn't have what it takes to win.

No wonder some of us with fewer resources and more chronic problems fail so routinely. You try to stuff the giant pillow of your problems into a small cardboard box labeled "FIXED," and just as you're tucking in the final corner, out pops another.

Or the same old one.

August 11, 1994

Long-haul conversations

This week I heard about an ugly accident in Washington, D.C., after a car ran a stop sign while the driver and his passenger were copulating.

I thought: What a waste of good drive time.

Beds are best for copulation.

Cars are best for conversation.

And nothing's better for a relationship than a long, long drive.

Locked together in a fast-moving vehicle, couples with several hundred miles ahead of them can discuss, explore and even — if the trip is long enough — resolve thorny issues like where to take their next vacation. Or what color to paint the sun porch.

Or whether to stay together.

The advantages of car talk: Neither party can escape. You sit within touching distance, but may easily avoid looking into each other's eyes.

And time is bountiful. With so many hours looming, even reluctant talkers often conclude that conversation is better than watching trees pass by.

My husband and I are pros at long hauls and marathon talks. Last weekend, we drove 20 hours to and from Washington. This weekend, we're on a 18-hour round-trip drive to Rochester, N.Y.

We're cheap, see. We'd rather spend $100 on gas and buy ourselves a hearty truck-stop dinner than hand $700 to an airline. Besides, you can hardly whisper on a plane without the guy in the other seat casting sidelong glances at you.

In a car, you can shout. You can cry. You can scowl. You can snort. About the only thing you ought not do is tickle. Or copulate.

Some of our highway conversations have been so involved that we've been startled to find we're rolling on fumes. Once we missed an essential exit on the Ohio Turnpike and drove an hour out of our way to get home.

And once the conversation grew so emotional that my husband pulled into a parking lot in Windsor and refused to cross the Ambassador Bridge unless we agreed to stop talking about the issue on which we had spent the last seven hours.

Now, of course, I can't remember what it was.

For those of you who might be starting long drives today, or anticipating one in the future, here are some tips.

■ One way to avoid conversation: Sleep. But whenever I hear that a couple spent a long drive just driving and sleeping, I think, "Uh-oh."

■ Good conversations often start with good questions. One of my favorites, useful in all circumstances: "So how have you been feeling about our life together?" Or, less ominously: "Tell me how your work has been going lately."

■ Some conversations get emotional. When one of you — especially the driver — begins to cry, it's best to pull over at a rest stop, fetch some Kleenex and coffee and chill out.

■ Other conversations turn silly. Don't be surprised if you start spinning fantasies for your future: you growing herbs, your partner raising goats. Or both of you selling everything you own and moving into a teepee in Saskatchewan.

■ Expect, too, to make lists. Of people you'd like to invite for dinner. Of fix-up jobs before your mother's visit. Of foods to cut out of your diet forever.

■ Some talks can't help but end wistfully, a little sadly. You've been talking for hours and see no resolution in sight. Dusk is falling. You've got two more hours before home. And you're tired. Too much, it seems, has already been said.

Then it's best to reach over and take your partner's hand, hold it tight and finish your drive in silence, watching the trees pass by, without letting a single word come between you.

May 28, 1993

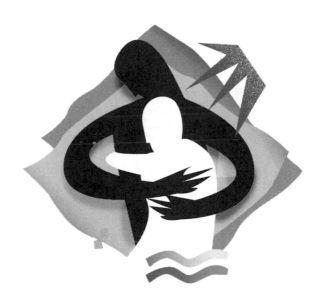

DOMESTIC RELATIONS

For want of a nail

When dusk arrived in my grandparents' house, we squinted. "Electricity is expensive!" my grandma would bark as our faces fell into shadows.

Grandpa made plenty of money working 43 years as a tool-and-die maker for Ford's. But he was not the family treasurer. Grandma believed money was for hoarding.

She did it well. Everything they owned was old and chintzy, nothing worth anything. Mom and Dad would buy them new pajamas or sweaters or belts, then years later find those gifts untouched in a closet, the tags still on.

Candy was easier and more reliable: They always ate it.

For a long time I considered them hollow people, empty of desire, content to sit in the dark in their little house on their threadbare furniture and indulge in a dish of vanilla ice cream before bed.

Grandpa, though, took some delight in tiny things, I knew. He noticed the lush flowers in my mother's yard, literally smacked his lips over her apple pie a la mode, and admired out loud the wistful tune of her wind chimes.

For his 85th birthday, I bought him small chimes — $60 cheaper than Mom's. But they made a tinkle so high-pitched that his hearing aid registered nothing. I swung them before his eyes, but he looked so blank and defeated that I cursed myself for causing him pain.

Two years ago at Thanksgiving I asked Grandpa what he wanted for Christmas. I expected indifference. Instead, instantly, as if he'd been waiting to be asked, Grandpa said: "I'd sure like a horseshoe nail. I haven't seen one in 75 years."

He looked away from us, as people do who are gathering memories. Then he told us about the mules he tended as a kid, working at the coal mine that later collapsed on his father and killed him.

I had never heard of horseshoe nails. For all I knew, you secured a horseshoe with the same nails you used to hang a picture. I called saddle shops, but they sold nails only in lots of 1,000. Finally, a brainstorm.

On a blizzardy morning, I drove to the Detroit Police Mounted Section near the Fisher Building and told the cops of my grandpa's oddball request. They laughed, but I left with three horseshoe nails, free from the City of Detroit.

I tied them with red ribbon and wrapped them in a little white cardboard jewelry box. On Christmas Eve, as we circled the room opening our gifts, I felt edgy as Grandpa's turn approached.

Perhaps he'd forgotten his request. Maybe he wouldn't recognize the nails — flat along one edge, with a ridged, triangular head. Or, maybe he'd been joking, and would be disappointed to get three nails instead of two dozen chocolate pecan turtles.

Awkwardly, he pulled the paper from the package. His hands, cramped with age, trembled to open the little box. He lifted the lid.

"Oh ho ho ho!" he cried, exultant. He clenched the nails in his bony fist and held them triumphantly to his face, as if they were the keys to immortality. "Oh, you kids," he said, with tears in his eyes, and, "I'll treasure these forever." All evening he cradled the box in his lap.

That night, before Dad drove him and Grandma home, I asked Grandpa what he'd like next year. He needed only a moment: "A bottle of wine from the Titanic."

For months the notion flickered through my head to find something from the Titanic, some relic, a button or a coin, although I suspected it would be fantastically expensive. I had no idea where to look, though, and I never got around to trying.

Last Christmas, I think, we gave Grandpa candy.

Two months ago, Grandpa said out of the blue: "I'd sure like a motorcycle ride before I die." I thought: How slow we are to learn each other's simple, silly longings. And I thought: I can make that happen.

Then I filed it away.

Last month, when he died, my dad found among Grandpa's few things the little white cardboard jewelry box. Grandpa had marked it SAVE in big black letters.

He never rode a motorcycle. He never sipped Titanic wine. He never told us all the other things he must have wanted, because we never asked.

We buried him in an old but adequate sport coat, a new belt around his waist, three horseshoe nails in his pocket.

October 12, 1992

Not to Ben & Jerry's taste

Dear Ben & Jerry:

You may soon receive a letter from my father suggesting that he be named the new CEO of your ice cream company now that you, Ben, are retiring at the frisky age of 43.

I urge you: Please reject him.

My dad, a little older, has been thinking about retiring, too, rooting around in his imagination for something to do after he no longer has to do anything.

He reads the paper line by line, so I'm sure he saw the news about your open competition for a new CEO.

Dad can't type, and his handwriting is illegible, but I figure he sent you a note anyway.

I can guess what he might have said. You announced the company now needed an "experienced CEO," so I imagine Dad reported he has lots of experience with ice cream and has been chief executive officer for 40 years of a household that has never gone bankrupt, shows a decent return on its investments, keeps an immaculate fleet of cars, believes in participatory management and which has never fallen victim to a takeover attempt.

I concede this: He's a big-hearted guy, fair to friend and foe, who's fun to work with and who would likely double everyone's vacation time, including his own, within his first week on the job. You might be able to survive that production dip, and many of your employees might enjoy the hammocks Dad would install at each work station. And it probably doesn't matter that my dad prefers straightforward ice cream names that tell you exactly what you're getting into — Butter Pecan, Strawberry — and has no clue why you choose the names you do. ("Cherry Garcia? Is that some Mexican fruit?")

But I want to warn you, there's more worth knowing:

■ First, he would compromise your ice cream every day.

He likes it melted. Lukewarm cream. He dishes it out, lets it sit for 10 minutes on the kitchen counter until it's soupy around the edges, then he slurps it up with his spoon as if it were split pea soup.

I also suspect that when he's alone, he licks the bowl, which might, because it demonstrates a childlike enthusiasm, be a PR plus.

■ Next, while I know you guys pride yourselves on creative flavors, you would be hard-pressed to find a market for the flavors I suspect he'd like to create: Watermelon With Salt. Banana Peanut Butter. Ice Cold Beer.

■ Last, if you chose my father as the next CEO of Ben & Jerry's Ice Cream, my mother would leave him.

My mother cannot control herself with ice cream. It tempts her more than Dad does. She lets it into the house only on rare occasions, then suffers each time she passes near the freezer. She swears she can eat a half-gallon at a sitting if no one is looking, and while you guys only make pints, I'm sure she could eat a few of those just as shamelessly. If my Dad were CEO of Ben & Jerry's, my mother would be fat, or gone.

So please, if you know what's best for your company and my family, send Dad a polite rejection letter, although a lifetime supply of half-off coupons might be a nice consolation.

June 28, 1994

The carnal competition

When on my answering machine I heard her voice, for the first time in 12 years, I remembered the weirdest things about her:

How she drank too much vodka at one workday lunch but slept it off beneath the sinks in the ladies' room.

How her husband, an accomplished attorney and quick conversationalist, routinely fell asleep at dinner parties.

And how once she told me that despite his propensity to naps, and six years of marriage, and a small child, they managed to make love every night.

I returned her call with trepidation. I knew she would ask what's new.

I've worked for the same company and lived with the same man for a decade. The sofa's even older. We have no new dependents, human or otherwise. I've taken up neither a foreign language nor yoga. I've given up meat, but who cares? I can now bake a loaf of bread that rises and I'm lately addicted to avocados. I've noticed a new line on my throat that seems permanent.

Is any of that "news"?

"So how are you?" I asked with enthusiasm, hoping she'd pick up the cue and not return the question.

What's new in her life is that her firstborn is now 14, a very talented violinist, first-ranked on her tennis squad and fluent in French, which her mother taught her. Her second-born is 10, a thoughtful and sensitive girl. And her third-born, a boy, is 2 and just starting to wend his way about the house.

Her husband is more accomplished than ever and commutes each day by subway to his work. Her own freelance career thrived until she quit a few months ago "to live," as she put it, "instead of work."

I could feel my spirit twitching as we talked. I definitely did not want to spend many minutes trying to inflate my own life.

So I popped right in with the main question on my mind:

"Hey! Do you still make love every night?"

I couldn't believe I dared to ask it, but I heard her laugh, so I figured it was OK, that we were communicating on the same intimate level we once did.

"Almost every night," she replied. "It's harder now with a 14-year-old who knows what's going on, and a 2-year-old who wants to be in the middle of everything. But there are still plenty of closets. And the bathroom."

I wanted to lie and say, "Ditto for us! Almost every night!" Instead I said, "Well, good for you," and meant it.

That night, I climbed into my same old bed with my same old man. And I told him about the phone call.

"They make love almost every night," I said, sighing.

"What does that mean?" he asked, and I realized I didn't know.

I didn't know what "making love" meant to them — who did what, for how long and who felt how when it was over. Normally a fearless interrogator, I had failed to ask the important follow-up questions.

My husband laughed at me. Then he said, "Probably their standards are very low." I smiled and remembered why I still loved him and we curled up together in our same old way and went fast to sleep.

November 28, 1993

My battered husband

Beneath his shorts my husband is hiding an incredible secret. It is 13½ inches long. It is 7 inches wide. It is the color of eggplant.

It is growing.

And we are paying it rapt attention.

It is the biggest bruise either of us has ever seen. A bruise the size of a platter. A bruise so huge I wince to see it but can't avoid it because there it is, on his upper left thigh, throbbing indigo.

We've gotten more laughs from it than from anything else recently, which makes me wonder if there's something very wrong with us.

I photographed it the other day as he sprawled on our bed. We think we might use the photo as the centerpiece of our 1993 Christmas card.

We discussed photographing it each day until it disappears. Then we could mount the snapshots in order on a huge board, put a frame around the lot and sell it for $10,000 to the Museum of Modern Art. "Bruise in Transition," we might call it.

I wondered if we might win a mention in the Guinness Book of World Records, but my husband said, "I think Evel Knievel has the edge on me."

We thought about others, too, who have probably been bluer: Sumo wrestlers. Roller derby stars. People who fall off ladders.

My husband's tale is less dramatic. Leaving the house early one morning, he slipped on a patch of ice and THWOMP!

Later, in the emergency room where medical types were verifying he hadn't busted anything, a nurse said, "I didn't think it was icy this morning."

Dead-panned my husband: "It was where I stepped."

For several days the bruise behaved itself, glowering in place.

Then, one morning, I couldn't believe my eyes: Overnight it had grown, migrated down his leg and across his groin. "Oh my God," I said, thinking gangrene, thinking amputation.

He went back to the doctor, who exclaimed over the bruise, but insisted he'd seen worse. A bruise is simply an accumulation of blood, spurted from broken capillaries, and the movement of that blood is normal, he said. Before the body reabsorbs it, he added, the bruise might roll all the way down his leg!

He says we are in for quite a show. The bruise will lighten a little, to a magenta color, then shift to a greenish yellow, all the while moving about as if my husband were a human lava lamp.

I'm still ashamed that I almost missed my husband's last big bruise. It was the size of a grapefruit, on his inner thigh, and it was 10 days old before I noticed it, which is shocking since we've been married eight years, sleep together every night, etc., etc. For weeks afterward, I felt a little blue about our marriage, that we could be battered and bruised without the other suspecting.

So we are pleased to watch this bruise together, as if we were lying on our backs beneath a summer sky, as fantastic animals and famous people's profiles appear and disappear in the shifting clouds. Last week we half expected to find, in its Lenten purpleness, a fuzzy face of Jesus.

Our life has rarely been so exciting. We awake in the morning with a new sense of purpose: checking on the bruise, remeasuring it (it grew to 2 feet long), exclaiming over its aurora borealis brilliance.

My husband still feels a little pain from the fall, but the bruise has won him pleasant attention. The women he works with inquire about it regularly, and even my mother has begged to see it.

He said no.

This bruise belongs to us.

April 14, 1993

Small, satisfying gifts

Since that first Christmas, when we exchanged our cheap little gifts in bed, we've worked harder to choose for each other bigger and better expressions of our love.

None has matched the first.

Each fall now, we protest that we want and need nothing that we don't already have. Yet, inevitably, a few weeks before Christmas, he or I will murmur before falling asleep, "Hey, I found you the perfect gift today." That compels the other to get busy.

One Christmas, afraid that my thrift suggested shrinking affection, I splurged and bought him a gorgeous $120 wool sweater.

He took it back. It made him sweat.

Another Christmas, he bought me big dazzling expensive earrings. I've found only one occasion to wear them, although they're beautiful in my drawer.

We continue this silliness, buying each other baubles and bathrobes and books, worrying they aren't right, aren't enough.

That first Christmas was easier.

We lived 2,000 miles apart. Our past was short and thin. Our future, who could say? We fantasized about one, though, a life rich with friends, conversation and food.

Our hopes weren't grand. We'd each been disappointed in relationships where the days were dull and, despite high anticipation, even weekends and vacations fell flat. All we wanted from each other was dailiness — the mundane satisfactions of companionship. Awaking in the same bed, sharing the details of our dreams, toast and coffee and the morning paper, reading the good stuff out loud. Going to our work with energy, finding a willing ear at the end of the day.

Then, cooking. Bumping buns in the kitchen, chopping, slicing, stirring. Making sauce and soup. Sitting down together for supper, like an old married couple.

Yet, that first Christmas, we were anxious, afraid to seem too eager, afraid to hope too much. We carried the small packages into the bed, where we spent a lot of our little time together.

He opened mine first: a garlic press, $2.49 I think it was, from Kmart.

Then I opened his: Two place mats, quilted cotton, in a simple blue-and-white pattern. Two matching napkins. From Pier One, he thinks. Less than $10.

We looked at each other. I remember a welling of pain. We had no home together. No table. No soup pot. No evening ritual. We shared only rare meals. These gifts, though, symbolized the daily life we might have.

Since then, we have done it. Mingled our things. Bought a home, then another. Shared meals first at his old butcher block table, then bought a new and bigger one.

Together we've eaten thousands of suppers. We've complained and cried, said mean and generous things, held each others' hands through individual and common troubles, wiped spaghetti sauce and blown our noses with our napkins. There have been nights when one or the other of us wasn't sure we'd make it to breakfast, or whether we wanted to. We've done everything at our table but start food fights.

Many new place mats have entered our home to sop up our spills.

But in our hutch, among the newer place mats, the old blue-and-white ones stand out. They are stained with who-knows-what, faded and frayed around the edges from hundreds of washings.

We pull them out on average Wednesdays, on blue Mondays, when one of us is feeling contrite or pensive, and on evenings when we come home surprisingly content and awed by the world. We set our soup bowls on those raggedy place mats, look across the table at each other, and remember that love is sturdy and daily, and that exactly this is what we wanted.

December 23, 1992

A daughter's belated regrets

Whose fathers does Hallmark know?
My dad's not like the dads portrayed on most Father's Day cards. For one, he doesn't own a duck decoy. Or a dog, or a boat, or a briefcase. He doesn't hunt or golf. He doesn't wear old-fashioned wire-rim bifocals, or drink whiskey from leather decanters.

Yes, he stands in front of a hot grill on summer evenings, flipping dinner. But he considers it a chore, not a hobby.

This year, as every year, there are no cards appropriate for my dad, who taught me many things but who, when I had the chance, I chose to slight instead of honor.

That slight is one of my life's regrets.

My mom and dad did not deliberate over baby-making as young couples do now. They just did it. So when my dad was 24, he had his first dependent: me. Within a few years he acquired two more children, a new $16,000 house and a role difficult to shrug off. He never tried.

Every Wednesday of my childhood, Dad loaded me and my brothers into the car and drove to the local library. While he waited, we knelt in front of the kiddie books, selecting a small pile. Dad perused and approved our choices, which was fine until I turned 13, wandered into the adult section, and began putting Mailer and Updike on my pile.

I'm not surprised that later, as teenagers, each of us kids took summer jobs at that library.

From my dad I learned to love books, and comfy armchairs, and good reading lamps. From Dad, too, I learned how a decent man treats a woman. Whenever he and Mom returned home from a big event, Dad would proclaim to us kids: "Your mother was the most beautiful woman in the room."

Dad also began a dinnertime ritual that still continues: rating my mother's meals with kisses. One kiss means OK, two means better, three is pretty darned good, four is excellent and five is outtathisworld. For as long as I can remember, though, no meal — even hot dogs and chips — has rated fewer than four kisses, which Dad administers loudly at the table.

From my dad I learned there's no such thing as a stupid question. From him I learned to try to make a joke when tension is rising between people, and to laugh at myself first. And from him I got my sentimentality. Whenever we sat as a family to watch a holiday TV special in which, for example, a prodigal son returns home at the last minute, Dad and I would use the most Kleenex.

So I wonder why, when I had my chance to recognize his influence on me, I didn't.

Because my father does not bully, whine or hold grudges, he never complained that when his firstborn child and only daughter decided to marry, she didn't ask him to walk her down the aisle.

Now, eight years later, I can't recall if I even explained my reasons to Dad: That a father "giving away" his daughter to a new man, as if either one owned her, seemed archaic, a holdover from centuries when men traded daughters for heads of cattle.

But mostly that, at nearly 32, I was my own woman.

Dad never said, "But what about me?"

So my partner and I walked down the aisle holding hands, while Dad stood in the front pew and smiled with tears in his eyes.

If I found a Father's Day card that said, "I'm sorry, Dad, for being such a damned feminist when I should have been a grateful daughter," Dad would read it and laugh, I know, and shrug and say "Oh, don't be silly."

Maybe I am being silly. But I think of how few opportunities for honor dads have in the lives of their children, and I regret that I didn't ask my father to join me for a few steps together on my wedding day.

That walk could have meant whatever Dad and I wanted it to.

June 18, 1993

Mother-daughter reflections

My polite and careful mother has grown more at ease with four-letter words. What trouble her now are words with three letters: "Old." And "fat."

My mother is not fat, but she worries it could happen. So she exercises daily in the basement on her treadmill or her ski machine or her bike, counting fat grams, weighing in each week as part of an inexpensive weight-loss program at which I suspect she is the slimmest one.

Neither is my mother old. Last week, she turned 63. But someone younger made a crack about her being old, and it stung, and she said to me, "I know I'm not middle-aged anymore, but I'm not old yet, am I? Why isn't there a word for what I am?"

And she said, "Getting older wouldn't be so bad if there weren't numbers attached."

Sympathetic, I wondered, "Who invented birthdays anyhow?"

Years ago, when calendars were scarce, nobody knew when they were born. You could grow older without knowing how old you were, in the same way you feel better in the morning if you ignored last night's clock and have no clue how few hours you slept.

In Mom's birthday card last week I wrote this quote from humorist James Thurber, who said in 1957: "I'm 63 and I guess that puts me in with the geriatrics, but if there were 15 months in every year, I'd only be 43."

If there were 27 months in each year, my mother would be only 28, which is what she feels like inside. Enthusiastic, idealistic, quick to pursue adventure, prone to sing while she works, eager for more. More of what? More of everything.

At 63, though, she looks out at the world through wiser eyes. Her legs have varicose veins now, which she hides well. She has to work harder to stay trim. She's more open-minded, more sure of herself. Imitating her own now-lost mother, she always looks terrific, even on her knees in the garden.

Since I was little people have said, "You look so much like your mother!" While that thrilled me at 8, I resented it by 18. No way did I want to look like Mom. When I was 23 and she was 45, we flew to New York City for a three-day fling, and even the desk clerk at the Waldorf Astoria noted our resemblance. Mom got a kick out of it. I wished I looked like myself.

In those early days of my womanhood, I found in my mail one day a quote from Shakespeare my mom had clipped from a magazine: "Thou art thy mother's glass, and she, in thee, calls back the lovely April of her prime."

As the years passed, I started glimpsing my mother's face in my mirror. At first I looked away. I was not ready for my prime to fade.

But now, I've reached some equilibrium. The winds of life are aging both of us now. I watch her face change, and my own, and I watch her sweat and pump that bicycle and slim down, as I plump up, and I think:

Oh, to be fat like Mom is fat.

Oh, to be old like Mom is old.

Oh, to hear someone say, "You look so much like your mother."

May 14, 1995

A relationship with no name

A wedding guest grasped my hand as I stood in the receiving line and beamed. "Congratulations!" he squawked. "Now you've got a daughter-in-law."

"Thank you," I said politely, then thought to myself, "Wait a second! I've never had a son."

Minutes earlier, my husband's son, Steven, had spoken all the classic vows that wed him until death to Brenda. She became my husband's daughter-in-law.

But what is she to me?

We laughed about it later: The language has dawdled so far behind social change no word describes what I am to Brenda, or what she is to me, or what Steven is to me, either.

When I met him 12 years ago, he was already 18. He has never called me anything but Susan. He introduces me as his dad's wife, and I introduce him as my husband's son.

We love each other, that I know. We love talking together, and teasing each other, dissecting recipes, discussing politics.

But I am not his stepmother. Because I am in the word business, we agreed long ago it's a poor word with a terrible reputation. Who's stepping on whom? Why are stepmothers in fairy tales always evil?

I am not his mother in any way. I did not mold him, although I like to believe that my affection, attention and questions — he teases me about my questions — have put some polish on his character.

I also suspect he has confided details of his life to me that he has not told his mother. Stories he would not have told me, probably, were I his mother.

At his wedding, his mother and I both stood in the first pew with tears in our eyes. But she remembered holding his tiny body in her arms, nursing him through colds and cuts and convulsions. I'm sure she remembered even the sound of his voice when he was 3.

I have memories, too, but I didn't give him life, or take care of him. Instead, we share feelings and ideas, no small things. Once we sat in the dark in the living room, with all the doors and windows open to the sounds and smells of a summer thunderstorm, and talked about his father, my husband.

Still, it seems there should be a word for me. Steven and his sister, Linda, don't make any particular point to call me on Mother's Day, which is fine by me, although once, early on, Linda sent me a homemade card that said "Happy Susan's Day."

I liked that. It was sweet and clever and suggested her own struggle to fit me into a role she could name.

When people ask, I tell them I'm more of an aunt to Steven and Linda than a mother, although even that falls short.

Most of the time, to tell the truth, I feel like a friend. Late on the evening of Steven's wedding, as he and his new wife and his sister and friends prepared to go out on the town for one last hurrah, I wanted to join them. I wanted to pack into a small car and smoke cigars and camp it up and win a free drink from some soft, sentimental bartender.

But we are not friends in the classic sense. We were thrust together by the choice their father and I made. We never chose each other as much as we chose to open ourselves to each other. To try, for the sake of their father and my husband, to love each other.

It worked, in time. Although no names exist for what we are to each other, we are committed to love and respect until death do us part.

And in time, who knows, having never been a mother, never been a stepmother, never been a mother-in-law, I may yet become a grandma, a role I think I can play and a title I think I can carry with grace.

What choice do I have?

November 16, 1995

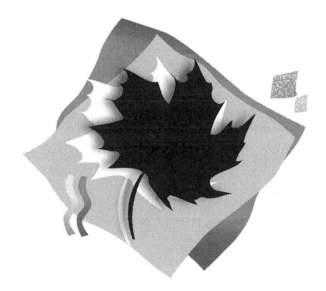

IN SEASON

Winter lets go of a cottage

The cottage in winter is stiff and cold.
We come to thaw it, and ourselves.

Nearly two feet of snow has fallen around it. We shovel for an hour to make a parking place for the truck. Then we shovel what has blown against the door and chip away at the ice until we can spring the screen door free and get in.

Inside, all is still and gray, the curtains closed tight against the light. A muted stench greets us. Somehow someone — probably me — left in the refrigerator a bag of brussels sprouts, some spinach, a pear.

A dozen insects lie dead on the floor. They disintegrate when I try to pick them up. Everything else is stiff, too: The sponge I used to wipe off the counter top in October. The bathroom towels crunchy with cold.

Inside the cupboards, the olive oil has clotted into green goop. The honey has turned white and thick. A can of mushroom soup is swollen.

We sigh and throw open the curtains.

Before us, 10 feet away, the frozen lake is white, blue, gray and awesome. We've never seen it like this.

We flick on the electricity, which includes baseboard heat. The cottage warms quickly because it is well-insulated and tiny. At 330 square feet — 30 feet long, 11 feet wide — it is twice the size of Thoreau's cabin at Walden Pond. But then there are two of us.

In winter, the cottage has everything but plumbing. Nothing flows in; nothing flows out. Everything must be carried.

My husband finds his winter boots, pulls them on and trudges to the lake to hack with an ax a hole through eight inches of ice.

We haul up washing water — storing it in buckets, heating it on the stove — and buy drinking water. We cook very little: Without tap water, cleanup takes too much time.

After our chores, we have a hard time loosening up. We feel edgy. Achy. Stiff. Unaccustomed to a place where the phone isn't ringing, the TV isn't yammering, nothing demands doing.

That night, after dinner out, we take our baths at the kitchen sink, standing on a rag rug, soaping ourselves up, squeezing the excess into a plastic slop pan, then stingily rinsing ourselves off, dripping onto the floor.

As I pour cupfuls of warm water over my head and into the pan, I remember a bath I took years ago while visiting a primitive Upper Peninsula cottage in winter with my boyfriend and his family.

After dark my boyfriend's father hauled a big tin washtub from a closet and into a bedroom. To fill the tub, his wife heated pot after pot of water on the propane stove. I watched, amazed and confused. Whose bath was this? And how deep into the night would this heating-and-bathing process last?

Then my boyfriend's father bowed to me and said: "Because you're the guest, you may bathe first." I suddenly understood: This tubful of water was everyone's bath.

Our kitchen sink baths are skimpier, but better. We don't have to share.

By the last morning of our stay, the cottage is thawed and snow is dripping from the roof. The refrigerator smells better. The dead insects are gone. Everything is fluffy, warm, inviting again. We listen to country music on the radio.

We walk for a long time on the ice along the shore, taking pictures of each other smiling and squinting against the brightness of snow and sky.

Then, before we leave and because it's 40 degrees, we take a real shower: out on the deck, sudsing up in the sun, pouring dishpans of hot water over our heads as steam rises off our skin.

We know that halfway home we'll start stiffening again. But as we pull away from the cottage, we look to the treetops and believe we see in them a faint blush of green.

March 24, 1993

Benign neglect and eggs

The hard-boiled egg earns the spotlight today when it's painted and prettied up. Naked, it's a plain and humble thing, but from it we can learn important life lessons.

First, some basics about eggs:

A white egg is no better than a brown egg. It's no different except for the color of its shell.

Why are some eggs brown and some white? Because some are laid by hens that lay brown eggs, and some are laid by hens that lay white eggs.

Inside, the eggs are the same.

I admire the egg's integrity. Intact in its fragile shell it cannot be injected with preservatives or artificial flavorings. You can't buy ranch-flavored eggs.

Because it does its job quietly, exactly as it has for eons, the egg is rarely recognized for the marvel it is.

The yolk of an egg comes together in a hen's ovary over several weeks. Guess how long a hen needs to build the white and shell around it.

Just 25 hours.

Every time you hold an egg in your hand, remember that, and allow yourself to be astonished. A team of engineers could not so swiftly construct such a wonder. Only a bird can. The average hen creates and lays about 275 eggs in her lifetime.

In my own life I've hard-boiled more eggs than that. I can't remember any very well, but I know some were too soft in the middle, and others had yolks coated in a dingy, unappetizing green.

I've used a timer, simmering them for 15 minutes, as my mother taught me. Then I tried 18 minutes. Then I tried turning off the heat and letting the eggs cook in the pan's hot water.

I couldn't rely on any of these methods. I never knew what I'd find when I cracked open my eggs.

Shouldn't following the rules guarantee success?

Turns out in eggs, as in life, no one best set of instructions exists. And no way works all the time.

I've figured this out about hard-boiling eggs: They turn out best when you don't care how they turn out.

Here's my current method: Put eggs in a pot with water. Bring to a boil. Keep boiling, or turn down the heat, or whatever. Ignore the eggs. Forget about them. When you remember, take them from the stove, set them in the sink and run cold water over them for awhile.

They will be easy to peel. And when you open them up you will see a perfect white and — this the amazing part — a perfect yolk, too. I am not teasing you. Fret less, relax more, enjoy your eggs.

Once, though, my husband and his first wife took this too far. One of them put eggs on to boil late in the evening and correctly forgot about them. They went to bed. They went to sleep.

Then boom! And boom! boom! They leapt up in alarm. In the kitchen they found an empty pot throbbing with heat on the stove, and 10,000 bits of hard-boiled egg splattered across the ceiling.

They spent that night on ladders with pails of sudsy water, scrubbing and scraping and being grouchy.

But they recall those exploded eggs more vividly than any other eggs they ever boiled.

That's a lesson, too: Failure makes a stronger memory than success, and a funnier story, too.

April 7, 1996

Wild in the berry patch

Nothing in life is free except wild black raspberries in July. Picking them will cost only a little time and a little skin.

Berry-picking is slow. You have to squeeze each one between your thumb and forefinger to ease it off. You can try to grab several at a time, but that won't work, or they'll get squished, and then you've got stains on your hands and probably your clothes, too.

The bushes are bristly. Your clothes will snag, and your arms and legs will get scratched, as if you played with a rambunctious cat. But the scratches only sting. They'll go away.

Other than that, wild berries are free. The black raspberry season is short, from about the Fourth of July to about now. I know this because a small patch grows a few yards from our house. Hundreds of people drive by the berries each day, but only a few of us pick them.

Among the pickers is my neighbor John, who first told me about them. He says he picks in the early morning, gathering a handful or two to sprinkle over his wife's cereal.

I like to go out at dusk, because it's quiet and still. I wade into the bramble on paths John has made. I reach for the most distant berries, the ones hidden behind leaves, the ones almost touching the ground, the ones in so deep that everything I'm wearing snags. I leave the easy berries for John, because he is twice as old as I, and because his wife will be waiting for her breakfast.

Country folk find free food all the time, I think. Nuts and berries and mushrooms and wild greens, edible flowers, flora I don't even recognize. We city folk have it harder. Our options: wild berries and black walnuts.

But black walnuts are a whole other story. If you know someone with a tree, they will inevitably offer to give you the harvest, which falls in early autumn, littering the lawn with nuts whose fleshy husks turn black and smelly.

Once, excited, I filled two black plastic garbage sacks full of nuts from some friends' backyard. I took them home, spread a tarp on the garage floor, put on my rubber duck boots and stomped all over them. Then I pulled rubber gloves over my hands to tug off the black husks.

My boots are still stained. So are the gloves. The tarp got tossed. The nuts eventually dried, but then it took half a day to crack them open, laying each nut on the sidewalk and smacking it with a hammer, picking tiny bits of meat out with a straight pin.

No fun. And when I finally baked a lemon and black walnut pound cake from my cup or so of nut meats, nobody liked it.

Do as you will, but my advice on black walnuts is to just say no.

Berries are easier. Even small-brained animals harvest berries, although which animals I don't know. I only pay attention to the bushes when I'm picking off them, thus scaring away other predators. But whatever eats the berries isn't efficient or greedy.

I am. Very greedy. Greedier about berries than about anything else in my life, because they're so bountiful. I could pick for hours, without gloves or rubber boots.

Usually, though, I stop after 15 minutes. While there's no such thing as a free lunch, in a quarter hour you can pick yourself a fine little dessert. With leftovers, even, for breakfast.

July 20, 1993

Plunge into summer

The bad news: Summer is half over.
The good news: Half remains.

By the calendar, of course, summer just started, with the year's longest day on June 21. But the rest of us know that the Fourth of July marks the season's psychic midpoint. As children we felt a touch of sadness as we stretched out languidly on the shady grass while Dad grilled burgers and Mom boiled corn: School seemed just around the corner.

Children are better than adults at squeezing the juice from summer, perhaps because they've known only a few. They haven't acquired that casual adult faith, "Oh well, if not this summer, next summer," that naive conviction that there will always be another.

If I knew this were my last summer, what would I do differently? An easier question: Would I do anything at all the same?

After work each day, I'd slide out of my hot clothes and put on my swimsuit and my flip-flops and run through the sprinkler, or walk to the neighborhood pool and dive right in, even if it were filled with noisy children. Instead of scowling when they splashed water in my eyes, I'd splash back.

I would wait till after dusk to walk home, relaxed and cool, thinking about nothing except the way the breeze felt on my wet hair.

I'd eat more watermelon, and not bother picking the seeds out first.

I'd buy the skimpiest sandals I could find, and not worry that my toes are funny-looking. Perhaps I'd paint my toenails, although I've never trusted women who do. I'd walk barefoot across the grass.

I'd get out of bed every morning at sunup, but first I'd move my bed into an east-facing room so the sun herself could rouse me.

I'd drink coffee each morning on the porch. I'd smear real butter on my toast, and I'd cut up bowlfuls of mangos and peaches and strawberries.

I wouldn't complain about rain. Maybe I wouldn't complain about anything.

Every evening I would grill my dinner, and during the rest of the day I'd eat only two kinds of food: wet or cold.

In the late evening I'd sit with the lights out and listen to the crickets.

I'd stay up to watch storms until the lightning faded.

I'd go to every free outdoor concert I could find, and when it took 45 minutes to get out of the parking lot, I'd roll down my window and ask the people around me how they had liked the show.

From the garage I'd pull down my old bicycle, and although its tires are now unfashionably narrow, I'd take it out one Saturday and pedal until I could pedal no more. That night I'd lie on top of my bedsheets smelling of Ben-Gay.

My bedsheets would be pure cotton.

I'd do all these things with the friends I've wanted to do things with, but never get around to. On long weekends I'd drive to see the people I've pledged for many summers to visit. On shorter weekends I'd go to the Potato Festival, and the Chicken Broil, and the Pesto Festival and all those corny festivals in all the small Michigan towns I can't find without a map. In each town I'd buy a Dairy Queen, and ask the clerks what they like best about living there.

Wherever I went, I'd take the time to suck each ice cube until it was gone.

July 5, 1994

Mama's special sauce

Family traditions begin this way:
Someone says, "Let's do what we did last year!" Then, "Let's do it again," and on and on, sometimes for decades, if a family is lucky.

Traditions end less neatly, often in fits and starts, fading, fading until suddenly there is no point in saving them.

The Cimino family of Dearborn Heights is at a turning point.

In late summer for 40 years, the Ciminos have made 100 quarts of tomato sauce, from a dozen bushels of ripe Roma tomatoes. The family's method, inefficient but familiar, employs, among other props, two white cotton pillowcases.

For decades before that the family's matriarch, Lidia Maria Cimino, made sauce as a child and young woman in Italy.

The procedure is so Old World that Mrs. Cimino still enforces a rule she learned in Italy: Any female who is having her period may not touch any tomatoes or come near the sauce, for fear it will turn green — a misfortune Mrs. Cimino swears she once witnessed.

For Mrs. Cimino (pronounced Chi-MEE-no), who is almost 71, tomato sauce is a lifetime tradition. But last year, she was too sick for the arduous process, which takes a day of intensive labor and several more days of preparation and cleanup.

This year, she's moving to a house a block from her only daughter. Her sauce-making equipment is packed away, and she will need some time to get her bearings in the new house. By then, tomato season will have passed.

Her three children and their spouses love Mama's sauce but generally dread the long, messy, sweaty process, in which each has a duty. "Who would ever ask their spouse to do all of this?" said oldest son Joe, who is 36.

So not one of her children picked up the tradition last year, or this year either. Joe rationalizes: "Mama is the foreman," and until she's back on the job, there's no point in a halfhearted — or half-informed — effort.

Packed somewhere in the cardboard boxes stacked in her house are what remains of the Cimino tradition: Six quarts of sauce, dated 1994, so few her children hesitate to ask her for even one.

"I am a little disappointed," she said to me in Italian and a bit of English, as Joe translated. "I wanted this year to make at least a couple bushels. The sauce is so good," she said, squeezing her fingers to her lips and kissing them.

"The jars you buy? No good."

With Joe's help, Mrs. Cimino described how she makes her sauce. Listening, you begin to wonder if maybe the no-good sauce you can buy from any store isn't good enough.

Each year about this time, Mrs. Cimino and other Italian women in her neighborhood placed tomato orders with a nearby fellow who drove to a farm in Ohio to load several dozen bushels of Romas onto his truck.

He delivered the tomatoes back to Dearborn Heights like an old-fashioned milkman, leaving them in garages, collecting about $10 per bushel. Joe and his brother hauled the bushels down the worn wood basement stairs, where their mother got on her hands and knees to spread hundreds of the small tomatoes onto blankets laid on the concrete floor.

Those already ripe were set to one side. Those still green were given two or three more days to ripen. Each day she checked: turning them, waiting, hoping to use every tomato she paid for.

Early in the morning on one of the first days of September, sauce helpers were assigned aprons: crisp white ones for those who handled the tomatoes, brown for those who handled just the jars.

The tomatoes were washed in a big colander in the laundry tub. Portion by portion, they boiled for half an hour in a huge blue speckled pot, so big only one can fit on the old stove in the basement.

The boiling separated the tomato skins from the meat, which someone scooped off the top and dumped into two heavy white pillowcases.

Each bulging pillowcase, oozing tomato juice, was twisted tight at the top, tied with twine, then hung from a metal pole extended between two chairs. For 45 minutes juice dripped from the pillowcases as those with the lowest status in the family squeezed and spun them, trying to force out every drop of liquid.

This, everyone agrees, was the worst job.

An old hand-cranked tomato mill sat on a table in the basement, the center of the action. Three times the tomatoes from the pillowcases were passed through this mill, making the sauce smoother and smoother.

Sterilized quart jars stood ready. Into the bottom of each was dropped a single bay leaf, and one or two leaves of fresh basil, which was earlier washed and air-dried on paper towel.

Mrs. Cimino poured the sauce into the jars. The men of the family tightened the lids.

Seven jars at a time were packed back into the same big blue pot where the tomatoes first cooked, and processed in boiling water for an hour.

That hot water was dumped. The pot was refilled with cold water, so not even a single cool new jar would crack, and another seven jars were processed for another hour.

And on. And on. The family took sandwich breaks upstairs — salami, mozzarella — but no wine and no heavy meal, "or else you'd never stand back up to go back down," Joe says.

Finished jars stood upside down on towels for still another hour, then all but one or two, which hadn't sealed well, were set in rows on the shelves of Mrs. Cimino's basement fruit cellar.

Then she cleaned up: mopping the basement floor, wiping splatters off everything, soaking the aprons and pillowcases in bleach for two days straight.

During its prime years, the Cimino family consumed two quarts of sauce each week. It was a foundation for many dishes.

Simmer it with ground veal, a little olive oil, fresh oregano and basil, and you had sauce for spaghetti, for example.

"She never cooked with a measuring cup," her son Joe says, "but with the hand and the tongue."

Since her husband died 12 years ago, Mrs. Cimino cooks much less and donates most of the sauce to her children.

But she knows how traditions die.

A good friend — one who lends her the tomato mill — is too sick to make her own sauce this year. The man who hauled the tomatoes from Ohio? He's had a stroke and won't ever deliver tomatoes again.

Her own mother used to make not just sauce but tomato paste — a harder job that required drying sauce in pots in the sun, stirring for days. Says Mrs. Cimino of that old tradition: "Forget it!"

But her own, she cannot dismiss, and neither can her children.

"As we get older and have families of our own," says Joe, "we look back and kind of miss what we had. For Mama, making tomato sauce these last few years made her feel more whole. It was that time of year we came together, and her house was full again."

Yes. She nods at his words as they sit at her kitchen table where once, every night, her whole family sat and ate her food.

"It's a lot of work, my sauce," she says. "Every year after I did it I would say to myself, 'I'm never going to make another jar.'

"But then you hear everybody talking about your sauce, how good it is.

"And you say: OK. One more year."

August 18, 1996

The naked truth

Summer's last gasp is over, and so is nakedness.
The house is chilly and at least the first half-hour of sleep feels better wrapped in flannel. But the very best kind of nakedness — in open air — is now impossible.

That makes me sad, because my favorite thing about summer is taking off my glasses, my shoes, my earrings, my top, my bottom, everything underneath and voila! I'm me again.

I'm no Madonna. I get no thrills from thinking someone will spy me naked, and don't think anyone ever has who didn't want to.

But, when I mention this to friends, nearly all smile wistfully and say, "Oh, I love to be naked, too." Makes me wonder if throughout our proud nation we all chafe each day within our clothes, and can't wait to get home at night to shed them.

I bet even Marilyn Quayle likes to be naked. Nakedness is as plain and wholesome as oatmeal cookies.

She probably goes to spas to be naked, though, or lounges on her private balcony, on guard for paparazzi. Me, I just step into my yard, which backs up to a woods, with the morning paper and a cup of coffee. Or, at the cottage, I pad to the end of the dock at dusk to watch the stars come out.

Is there anyone on earth who wouldn't rather be naked, alone and secure under a warm sun, than swaddled in clothes?

Yes, an old boyfriend of mine. We liked to drive through the hills north of San Francisco. And I liked to stop, grab the blanket from the trunk and wade through the tall grass to a private spot where I could lie on my back for a few minutes, with nothing between me and the sky.

He would wait in the car, and look embarrassed when I got back in.

Once, we went camping in the mountains, miles from anyone.

Everywhere we looked was rock and ridge and light and shadows and emptiness. The first evening, I kept my clothes on, for his sake, until we got into the tent. But the next morning, exploring, I felt so awed by that spot and, I guess, by the wonders of life in general, that I suggested we take off our clothes and just stretch out like children on one of those huge slabs of rock.

He said no.

So I lay there alone. He sat on the next rock fully clothed, his hands folded in his lap, until I sighed and got dressed.

How cruel of me, you say. He must be insecure about his body.

No, I think he liked his body plenty. I did, too, even though it was thin and white and goosebumped like a plucked chicken. In the privacy of his own place, he loved to be naked and prance like John Travolta in "Saturday Night Fever."

Still, if he were insecure, nakedness might have helped. Nakedness buoys me, especially when I'm feeling doughy and dumpy. You see your naked body often enough, especially under sunny skies, and you grow accustomed to its ripples and dimples and oddities.

It becomes yours — like the face you see in mirrors every day and which you don't hesitate to show to strangers.

I smile when I hear about the bold women in Toronto and Rochester, N.Y., who regularly march bare-breasted through the streets to demand equal nudity rights. I suspect we'd all be happier if we could be naked more often, and in more places.

But I'd never march. That turns nakedness political. And mine isn't.

It's the exhilaration of being, for a few minutes, just a creature: no props, no pretensions, nothing separating my skin from the rough wood of the dock, or the dew on the Adirondack chair, or the scratch of a wool blanket while, overhead, the geese fly south.

October 16, 1992

A gray month has its gifts

On a day as dreary and irredeemable as a wet newspaper, I went down to the basement to roll socks.

His socks. His hundred-and-one socks, all shades of navy and black. I had to squint. I had to lay them out and measure them against each other, and scrutinize the texture, and make judgments.

Finally, I carried the dozens of rolls in my arms up the stairs to his sock drawer.

There's no punch line to this story except that after rolling those socks, I felt better than before I began. As I knew I would.

Only two things are worse than the November blues: the February blues (poets tend to kill themselves in this month), and the absence of any reliable blues-buster, however temporary.

The season is ruthless. When I was at Michigan State I found, in a student literary publication, a little poem that I never wrote down but never forgot: "Just when you think you've forgotten
the tragedies of autumn,
a leaf touches upon your shoulder
like a tiny hand."

Some people I know can only wallow, wrapping their melancholy around them like a cloak, skulking through their days. They're not clinically depressed; they're just helpless.

One friend says of this month: "Yeah, it's my worst. I keep thinking if I die, it'll be in November. I feel inadequate, insecure, old, unloved. You name it. If I still drank, I'd be deep into wine."

Instead, he buys Christmas gifts, way early. Or he gives money away. This is the same friend who once advised me, when I was numb with ennui, to 1) buy some art, nothing too expensive, 2) see a totally mindless comedy like "Road to Morocco," 3) visit a soup kitchen or 4) visit Home Depot.

All good blues-busters. Other people I know do a crossword

puzzle, build a fire, clean off a desk, or play a silly game with a silly child.

The man whose socks I rolled swears by White Castle. Sliders from the freezer zapped in the microwave are insufficient. He must get in his car and drive to the White Castle and sit there and hear the sizzle and inhale the grease while he eats.

For me, baths are a cheap, quick fix. Better is when I can take with me into the tub a ridiculously expensive bar of soap.

But the other day when the blues struck, I was at the office. No tub around. No unoccupied socks.

So, I put on my coat and took a walk. To help my mood, I tilted my face toward the sodden sky to catch whatever dribble of light might penetrate the clouds.

I stood on a corner as a young man in a wheelchair navigated with his one good arm. He wore bright yellow leggings.

I watched as an enormously fat woman in a brilliantly green coat crossed the street.

Near Greektown, a woman who was lost asked me for directions. A man half my age stepped up, too. Together we were able to help her find her way.

In a pastry shop, I overheard a pretty woman tell her companion that she had already lost 30 pounds. They each bought a sugar-free chocolate peanut butter candy, 25 cents apiece.

I selected a dozen pastries, $9 worth, each one different. I took my time choosing them, imagining how each would taste in my mouth.

But I'm only one person, so when I got back to work I set aside a cannoli for myself, then walked the box around. "What's the occasion?" people exclaimed.

Within two minutes, the box was empty. I was full again. And I remembered my middle-aged, November-blue buddy and E-mailed him: "Want half a cannoli?"

He replied: "Nah. It'd kill me."

November 13, 1992

With grim gratitude

Thanksgiving is my favorite holiday: It demands no huge expenditures, can fly with only a bit of planning and focuses unabashedly on optimism and food.

The trouble with Thanksgiving, and its abiding challenge, is that sometimes it comes when we feel least inclined to gratitude.

The deepening gray of November turns our spirits soggy with old memories of better times. While Thanksgiving is about counting our blessings, anyone who has lived a few years has figured out that blessings are fleeting. Health fades, and so, too often, does love. The grand old tree that graced a yard for a century loses its sap and its vigor, and it, too, is lost to us.

Life's raw facts are hard: Inevitably, we lose what we love. If nothing else, we lose our balance and our youth. We lose our way, or our rhythm.

The blessings of one harvest season are the regrets of another. Harder to remember is the flip side, the truth that keeps us going: From the sadness of one year spring the blessings of the next.

I remember a Thanksgiving dinner at our place a few years ago. At a long rented table, covered with a big green rented tablecloth, sat my three living grandparents. Two are gone now, and the last is frail and confused in a nursing home. But new at our table this year will be my brother's partner's little boys, ages 5 and 6, bubblier and more fun, I have to say, than the grandparents ever were.

At that past Thanksgiving, we took turns saying what we were most thankful for. One friend looked into his wife's eyes and exalted their love. Another couple tearfully thanked God that finally, after years of effort, they were five months pregnant.

The marriage so lavishly praised ended within a few months — her idea. The baby so eagerly anticipated died before it could be born.

This Thanksgiving, although their loss has not faded, my friends have two bright, beautiful children they've adopted.

My abandoned friend found a new wife, and the woman who left him is working at a new job, feeling better than ever about herself.

And I'm thinking about the couple in Chicago whose six children were killed two weeks ago in a freeway fire. My first instinct: They cannot sanely celebrate Thanksgiving this year.

But on TV I watched the father, his face scabbed over with burns, say he was thankful his children died instantly. And, he said, "We understand that trials come. If our faith is not tested, then it is empty.

"We will laugh and smile with tremendous memories of our kids."

His serenity took me by surprise. But then it seemed right and healthy. It reminded me of a favorite line about loss, from May Sarton's classic "Journal of a Solitude." "I think of the trees," Sarton wrote, "and how simply they let go, let fall the riches of a season …"

So few of us can do that. We want to keep and hold onto everything good. It makes us crazy that life is about as many good-byes as hellos.

Would that we could let go without clutching, and open our arms with faith to what new blessings await us, if not this Thanksgiving, then next.

November 22, 1994

A holiday letter worth reading

I t's not too late to compose a Christmas letter that tells your friends what they really want to know about your year.

Skip the gushy descriptions of your Caribbean vacation, your bright children's excellent report cards and the new porch you built so you could invite your neighbors for iced tea and fellowship.

Nobody cares how many flowers you had on your peony bush, or that you discovered your great-great-grandfather's grave, or that you glimpsed Bill Clinton on his morning jog while you were in Washington on business.

Here's what they do care about:

■ How much money are you making?

■ What kind of exercise do you do? If you jog, do you have that little twinge in your knee, too? Can you bend over and touch your toes 100 times? What sort of excuses do you use to avoid exercise?

■ How many Dr. Scholl's foot products have you purchased this year? Be specific.

■ How much do you weigh now? What's to blame? How much have you eaten in one sitting, and what brought on that binge? About what food habit do you feel most guilty? Be specific. For example: "I love a spoonful of crunchy peanut butter dunked into the jar of Hershey's chocolate syrup."

■ How about sex? More or less than last year? More or less satisfying? Any new fool-proof gimmicks?

■ On a 1 to 10 scale, how's your primary relationship? What petty things do you still fight over? Example: "We're still together even though he leaves his empty cereal bowl sitting for hours in the sink until the little flakes are cemented to the sides." When's the last time the two of you laughed uncontrollably in bed? If it was over a joke, please do recount it.

■ What's the worst or weirdest health ailment you've suffered this year? Were you brave or did it make you feel like a helpless little child?

■ Did you love or hate "The Bridges of Madison County?" And if you haven't read it, go out and buy it before you write your Christmas letter, because the future of many friendships may depend on the answer to this question.

■ When you look in the mirror these days, which of your relatives do you see? Where on your face does most of your stress show up? Would friends you haven't seen in 10 years recognize you?

■What about your hair? Do you artificially enhance it in any way? Or have you given up? Did you even think about buying that funny spray paint for your bald spot?

■ What's the rudest thing each of your kids has said to you this year? The sweetest? How many times have you wished you were a cabaret singer in Paris instead of a mother in Muskegon?

■ Be honest: If you could, what time would you go to bed? How often do you lie awake in the middle of the night? What do you think about?

■ How many times this year have you spent all day in your pajamas? Did it make you feel sad or indescribably contented?

■ Over what did you cry this year? Do you feel better now?

■ What do you wish you'd done this year that you didn't? What do you want to do next year that you think you actually might?

■ Have you figured out the meaning of life? If so, please do recount it. Be specific.

December 12, 1993

Add one pinch of tradition

No one has ever asked for the recipe for my nut bread, from which I should take a clue.

But I don't. I bake it nearly every Christmas, and continue to call it mine, even though it's no more "my nut bread" than a carol I sing is mine or a sonata I play on the piano belongs to me.

Last year, thinking maybe it was too decadent for the '90s, I made a low-fat pumpkin bread instead.

Nobody asked me for that recipe either. Worse, the bread was too easy. It felt like a capitulation to convenience.

I missed my nut bread ritual. So this year I revived it. Each morning I'm getting up a few minutes early to baste my breads in marsala, a dark, sweet, fragrant wine. I stand groggy at the kitchen counter in my sweats, awash in coffee and marsala and memory. I unwrap the loaves from their foil and cheesecloth and brush them — bottom, sides, top — with the wine, then refold the foil and return them to the fridge.

From my cookbook notes, I can see I've made the bread at least since 1984, when I tripled the recipe to get 10 small and 7 medium loaves. The ingredients that year — including 21 cups of pecans and walnuts — cost only $24.82.

I guess I make my nut bread for the same reason my Great-Uncle Stanley, at 83, continues to climb all over his little house in Detroit hanging Christmas lights. He doesn't do it for the admiration of the neighbors, most of whom have died since he bought the house in '65. He doesn't know the new people. His wife, Aunt Helen, complains about the strands all stuck in one plug, which sometimes blows a fuse.

Uncle Stanley hangs his lights because he always has, and because he still can.

In Dearborn Heights, my mother is packing 200 frozen pierogi into Tupperware boxes to transport to Minnesota for our Christmas Eve feast at my brother's. She made 350 but will keep some at home to spice up humdrum winter dinners with my dad. This year she worked for 12 hours over two days on five varieties of the Polish dumplings.

She will make those pierogi each Christmas until she can no longer stand. Then one of us will take over, or dare to suggest some other delicacy, although a new idea substituted for an old ritual always feels raw and lonely.

Meanwhile, in Florida, my mother-in-law is baking her famous Christmas wreath cookies. They are simple: a sugar cookie flavored with anise and cut in the shape of wreaths. Never bells or stars. Only wreaths, frosted in green and dotted with red cinnamon candies.

Her grandchildren, my husband's kids, used to beg for and gobble her wreaths. Now they are grown and far away at Christmas, too busy and distracted to bake those cookies.

But she still does, in memory of what they used to mean.

Time rushes on, carrying us with it. Each holiday a different set of people gathers around our tables, and even if their faces are the same, their hopes and fears have changed.

Death steals some of them. So does life. Because we can't control much, we cling to the details, the little things we are capable of repeating over and over, that help us remember who we were and still are, that root us in our place, that save us from being blown hither and yon by the wind.

December 21, 1993

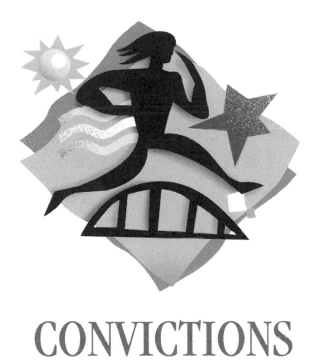

CONVICTIONS

Bagels, lox and wisdom

In this season of goodwill, when even those we love act erratically and nobody cooperates as they should, I have a parable.

It is a parable of our times, although it happened to me many years ago, when I was a student at Michigan State University and a member of the student newspaper staff.

From this episode, I gleaned one of the most valuable bits of wisdom from my years at MSU. Oh, sure, I learned not to mix Black Russians with even the smallest sip of tequila. And I learned that when you get home exceedingly late, it's best not to look at a clock. You will feel better the next morning if you think maybe you got four hours of sleep instead of two.

But this wisdom is stronger. I've carried it and used it in my life as a professional journalist and a full-time human being. It has buoyed me during many dark nights of the soul, and many Christmases.

It may help you, too.

Or it might make you feel worse about everything.

In those days we typed our stories on clunky, noisy manual typewriters and corrected them with fat black pencils like kids use in kindergarten. Editors added more pencil marks, then rolled my stories and everyone else's together into bundles, securing them with rubber bands.

Somebody had to carry these bundles to a composing room a few blocks away, where the words were set in type, then pasted on a newspaper page along with headlines.

The carrying of story bundles to the composing room was called a "copy run," and the chore went to whoever wasn't busy with something else.

Lo, there soon appeared on the copy run path a new shop selling bagels of all varieties, spread with all sorts of cheeses and goops.

Soon every copy run included a bagel run.

The runner would circle the newsroom, taking orders, writing them on a scrap of paper. The runner would dash the few blocks to the composing room, then fetch the bagels on the way back.

One day, being the runner, I found myself in an exceedingly long line at the bagel shop, longer than I'd ever seen, spilling out onto the slushy sidewalk. Everyone in line was muttering. They had places to go! Things to do!

So did I.

As the line inched into the shop, I realized the problem: Only one worker was filling orders. Three others who would normally be up front too were instead loafing in the back room, visible to all of us, chatting it up and smoking and laughing and having a great time.

Filling our orders and taking crap from everyone in line was a mousy fellow, frail, pale, with thin reddish hair. I would recognize him today.

He did not rush. He methodically split and buttered bagels, laying lox or spreading tuna on top, wrapping them in paper, hardly looking up from his tedium, never reacting to the insolence of those who had to wait so long.

Finally, I reached the front of the line. I couldn't help exploding at him, not over my wait but over his passivity.

"How can you stand this?" I hollered. "Here you are taking abuse from all of us while your coworkers refuse to do their jobs!"

Startled, he looked up from his work, a spatula filled with cream cheese in his hand.

Then he said these words, words I've said to myself time and again in the decades since, whenever I'm out of my mind with worry or anxiety or rage.

He shrugged and said: "What will it matter in 10,000 years?"

The moral of the story: Do the best you can, given the circumstances. Ignore the jerks around you. Maintain serenity.

December 21, 1992

News expands our world

A local attorney tells me he has no time to read newspapers, can't stand the "shooting and slashing" on TV news, and gathers news of his neighborhood and his world the old way: by word of mouth.

If an event triggers talk in the barbershop or cafeteria, he hears of it. If it doesn't, he never misses not knowing.

By his standard, the only recent news involved Tonya, O.J. and the big LA quake.

A bystander to my chat with the attorney asked: "From whom did you hear about the rivalry between the Hutus and the Tutsis?" The bewildered attorney's brow furrowed. He had not heard enough about the massacre in Rwanda to know the names of its tribes.

When we explained, he shrugged. "I don't need to know that."

Who could disagree? But is "need to know" the only reason we should suck on the news?

I've known days when I didn't want to hear one more account of one more pitiful situation in one more pathetic nation I'll never visit. We all have.

The claustrophobia of my own concerns is cured, though, by considering others'. To live in a larger world is to breathe fresher air.

What happens to a person who turns off the radio, the TV, the newspapers and lives day after day without any news of places more distant than the corner intersection?

That person shrinks. While a resident of the world, the person without news cannot be a true citizen of it.

Years ago I loved such a man. He called himself an intellectual and read fat books. Our conversations were vigorous, but we talked about abstracts. He cited few facts to support his opinions. He told no tales to illuminate his points.

Plus, he viewed life as simple — right and wrong, good and evil.

I did not believe that. I had read about quandaries with no resolution, questions with no answers and people behaving in inexplicable ways.

Worst of all, he never voted, because he never knew enough to care enough to want to make any difference.

How could I love him? I was young.

More recently, I shared an uneasy dinner with my stepson and his then-girlfriend who, before the cheese melted on our spaghetti, started in on the media.

She, too, never consumes news. "It's all so many lies," she insisted, "intended to sell newspapers and advertising."

I should have been contrite for choosing such a slimy career. Instead, I felt sorry for my stepson, who slurps news with gusto, digesting it out loud and in the privacy of his own head.

That's its point: to provoke thought and talk. Each day's news is another layer of lemon peels and carrot scraps on a compost heap. The pile may smell, but from it comes healthy soil in which good things grow.

Citizens of the world don't read newspapers to learn the truth, because the truth is slippery. Facts change. Suppositions collapse. Assumptions explode. Mistakes are made, and newspapers must sometimes correct themselves because someone's finger slipped on the keyboard.

People read and watch news in search of understanding, a pursuit that can keep anyone excited, engaged and enlarged for a lifetime.

July 31, 1994

Farewell, Richard Nixon

The day Richard Nixon resigned, I drank scotch for the first time, warm and neat from a wax-coated paper cup, in the Free Press newsroom.

I was 20 years old, an intern at the paper the summer between my junior and senior years at Michigan State. I was naive, in over my head every day. And like many of my peers, I had spent the previous year sick to my stomach about Watergate. Those long nights of putting out the MSU student paper, editing down the Watergate tapes, gave us a giddy glimmer of power — we, too, constituted "the press," chipping away at evil in the White House.

Yet in our bellies throbbed the same dread we knew as third-graders during air-raid drills, scrunched under our desks, our heads between our legs, wanting to believe this was just pretend, but suspecting bombs would fall any second and the school collapse to crush our heads.

On August 8, 1974, the day Nixon announced his resignation, I was among the youngest reporters in the Free Press newsroom. I remember a veteran newsman lugging a cardboard case of Johnnie Walker Red into the city room, setting it on an editor's desk and slashing it open with gusto and an Exacto knife.

When the moment came for Nixon's announcment, we packed our sweaty selves into the executive editor's office to watch the newsroom's only TV. Everybody whooped and cheered, lifting their paper cups of scotch in a toast to themselves and the process, while I stood squeezed against a back wall with tears in my eyes.

I felt sorry for Nixon, sorry that a man could rise so high yet be so arrogantly cavalier and foolish and cruel to those of us who, in our youth and sentimentality, counted on the president for security the way we had counted on our grade-school nuns, or our fathers.

The tears were cathartic, too. For so long I had felt so afraid. Our long national nightmare was over.

One woman I know, a regular at anti-war rallies, once gave the finger to Richard Nixon, but felt tears, too, when he resigned, and again when he died last week. We decided we must have seen in him an exaggerated version of our own awkward, geeky, pathetic selves: guilty of senseless transgressions against those who rely on us, but hoping through sheer willpower to win redemption and forgiveness.

Another woman my age watched Nixon's resignation on an old black-and-white TV in Stockholm with other U.S. exchange students. No cheers. No tears. Just dead silence. And, she remembers, a feeling that they and the rest of America back home had emerged "from a long dark tunnel, and were lying on the side of the road trying to catch our breaths."

Tomorrow, the first president of our generation will give an improbable eulogy for his predecessor who betrayed us. The nation will fly its flags at half-staff, as it does to honor heroes, for a man many Americans consider no more than a common, naked criminal who happened to wear, for a time, the clothing of an emperor.

Twenty years after that muggy August day when I sipped my first scotch, I still cannot drink scotch without remembering how terrible those last months of Richard Nixon were. When I mourn, I don't mourn him, but the faith my generation lost.

April 26, 1994

The unadorned Susan

My mother put mascara on my eyelashes the night of my senior prom, and years later insisted I wear lipstick on my wedding day.

Her argument is simple: Every woman looks better with a little makeup.

Mine is simple, too: I want to look like I look. I want my naked face to be my only face.

I aim for authenticity.

I came of age when many women scorned makeup and other female props. In college my buddies of both genders all dressed alike: jeans, flannel shirts, heavy socks, no earrings, no makeup.

But then my friends graduated into the real world, buying suits and ties, pumps and panty hose. Women woke up to rub sleep from their eyes, then add mascara and shadow and liner.

I capitulated to femininity in a few small ways, including earrings and bras. But heels were no good for covering fires or climbing up embankments to train wrecks. And I refused to wear makeup, on principal, even when winter turned my face sallow.

People who are different, by fate or choice, maintain their self-esteem by finding some small advantage in their dissimilarity. At parties I imagined all the beautiful lacquered women to be hollow inside. I imagined men drawn to my face because I hid none of it.

I did not need a mirror in my purse. I did not leave stains on wine glasses.

All this was hooey. I was no less insecure and no more alluring than any other woman. By the time I turned 40 I stopped defining my cosmetic-free face as some badge of honor, but wore it comfortably and without much thought.

Then something terrible happened.

A few days ago, I got a professional makeup job. A woman

named Annie devoted 30 minutes to my face, preparing me for a TV commercial in which I would promote the Free Press.

When she was through, I looked in the mirror and, to my horror, I liked who I saw. She was ... pretty.

An epiphany thundered through me: This is how good you could have looked all your life if only you had tried.

I drove straight to my parents' house. Mom was thrilled. Dad would have taken pictures except the battery in his camera was dead. Even my husband acted impressed, and shot a dozen photos.

That night I washed off my new face with some regret. The next morning I scrounged through my drawers to find a freebie lipstick sample and an eyeliner my stepdaughter left behind and an old jar of something called Indian Earth, authentic red clay from somewhere out West that colors your cheeks.

For 15 minutes, in front of the mirror, I enhanced my face, awkward with the tools and sheepish about my sudden betrayal of principal.

That day at work, a guy I've known for years said, "I don't know what you're doing, but you look terrific."

I thanked him, but inside I groaned.

For a few more days I wore mascara and eyeliner and lipstick. I could feel it on my face, greasy, a little itchy. I needed frequent touch-ups. My face felt separate from the rest of me, preceding me wherever I went.

Stop this, I told myself, or you'll be sucked in forever.

The next day I shyly took my familiar naked face back to work with me.

Nobody said anything. My face won no compliments, but it didn't mind.

Ease is its own reward.

March 3, 1996

The tyrant within

This month marks the 29th anniversary of the most intimate, most uneasy relationship of my life.

I was a few weeks shy of 11 when I was diagnosed with diabetes, after a month of weight loss and fatigue so dramatic that I was two or three pounds lighter each day, and would stumble home from school, throw my book bag on the floor and fall into bed until dinner.

I had never heard of the disease the doctor said I had. But he told me it would be forever.

Thank God, at 11, I didn't realize how long that was.

My partner in life, diabetes has made me who I am, yet I hardly understand it. As old married couples will say, though, we've reached some accommodation, my disease and I. Problem is I'm the one who's done all the compromising. It never relents, never retreats.

I measure its mood several times a day with a $39 gadget that, after I've pricked my finger and squeezed out a drop of blood, tells me how far off normal my blood sugar is. A normal person, even after a hot fudge sundae, will register between 80 and 140. For diabetics, a handful of potato chips or the adrenalin of 20 minutes of high emotion will shoot the number to 200.

If my number is high, I inject insulin. If it's low, I eat carbohydrates. If it's normal, I sigh and wonder what I did right, knowing full well that other times when I do everything right the numbers are dramatically wrong.

The injections are the least of it. I now take five or six a day, usually in my abdomen, right through my clothes, often in public. But they're no more difficult or painful than brushing my teeth. The hard part of the disease is paying attention — every meal, every day, no vacations.

And the worst part is there's no getting away with anything. Sure, I cheat. Everyone does. A sliver of a friend's birthday cake, a few after-dinner mints, a foil sack of airline honey-roasted peanuts. But for every sin I pay a price within an hour: higher blood sugar, and a sick, thick, sluggish feeling. Over time, high and erratic blood sugar destroys the tiny blood vessels in the eyes and kidneys, and speeds up the hardening of arteries, dramatically increasing the risk of blindness, kidney disease, heart failure, loss of limbs.

Although I worry about each twinge and ache and skipped heartbeat, I'm fine so far. No complications except those of the spirit: regular vexation over sharing my body with an unreasonable, unyielding, unsympathetic bully. Then, though, I feel guilty for resenting a disease that has neither killed nor maimed me, but with which I've managed to build a life, albeit an idiosyncratic one.

In the same way that tallness or shortness or smarts or birthmarks thread their way through a child's developing personality, my disease served as a kernel for the adult I became.

Its possible threats to an unborn child scared me away from having any. I joined Zero Population Growth when I was 13, never fantasized about being a mom and am now content to be childless.

The rules and schedules by which I lived turned me into a rebel against almost all rules, regulations, expectations. A friend my age who is a 30-year diabetic carries the same trait. Her husband calls her "the rebel without a cause."

Because diabetics are prone to early death, I've never imagined living past my mid-50s. I resisted investing in an IRA because you have to be 59 to collect it. And I hate planning, even for vacations. For me, the future is uncertain and dark, so I cast my hopes with today.

Who would I be, I sometimes wonder, if it weren't for this disease? Do I control it, or does it control me? Alas, we alternate leading the dance. Maybe I attribute to it all the soft spots of personality that would have been there anyhow.

And yet, it's done me good, too.

I'm healthier than I would have been if I'd ranged freely and without limits through the aisles of my life's supermarkets.

I'm attentive to people and problems, I think, because I've learned that paying attention involves more than focusing now and again, but requires daily, even hourly commitment.

I'm resilient, having learned early that a good number will follow a bad the way a bad number will follow a good. I can't take a string of bad numbers personally, or I'll lose the energy to turn them around.

Chronic disease, I've learned, is best approached day by day, just like life. Each meal is a new chance to succeed.

Best, though, from my perspective, is that my diabetes has taught me to find more joy in food than anyone else I know.

When I was young and just diagnosed, my mother and captain of my diet would prepare my evening snack by counting 12 salted peanuts into a shot glass. I would separate the peanuts and suck each half until it disintegrated, thereby stretching my snack to last hours.

I'm still one to stretch my pleasures, to lick my plate. To try, whenever I can, to hold the hand of my disease and act as if we're friends.

January 25, 1993

The magic of three

No ifs, ands or buts about it: Three enjoys a magic and rhythm that two and four lack.

John and Michelle Engler will learn what preachers and writers already know: Three is powerful. Memorable. Dramatic. Two is tepid. Four is overwrought.

Three works.

Had the Engler triplets been boys, they might have been Larry, Moe and Curly. Or Winken, Blinken and Nod. With mixed genders, they might have been Peter, Paul and Mary.

The girls, by birth order, became Margaret, Hannah and Madeleine. Nickname two, and you've got a winning law firm: Hannah, Maddy and Meg.

Three is magical because we think about much of the world in contrasting pairs: men and women, body and soul, fire and ice.

Couples make the world go 'round, but trios give it zest: Men, women and children. Red, white and blue. Bacon, lettuce and tomato.

The musketeers were three. So were the blind mice and the Magi. So were the witches who chanted around a bubbling cauldron in "Macbeth."

The genie gave Aladdin three wishes. We give our friends three guesses. Realtors cite the three most important things to look for in a house: Location, location, location.

Animal, vegetable or mineral? Coffee, tea or milk? Children study readin', 'ritin' and 'rithmetic, and learn their ABCs — not ABs or ABCDs.

What's so wrong with two and four? Think about it geometrically: Two points make nothing but a straight line.

Mork and Mindy. Frick and Frack. Black and white.

Three points make a triangle, elegant and interesting.

The Father, Son and Holy Spirit.

The butcher, the baker, the candlestick maker.

A loaf of bread, a jug of wine and thou.

With four points, you get some variety, but four words or concepts are one too many for graceful recollection.

We can name the Beatles, but each of us chooses a different order. Same with the seasons. I start with winter. My husband starts with summer, because he remembers the "Howdy Doody" show and Princess Summerfall Winterspring.

Whoever named the rock group Blood, Sweat and Tears was wise to the magic of three. The name comes from a Winston Churchill pledge to end World War II with "blood, toil, tears and sweat," but I always have to look up that quote to remember the correct order.

Advice goes down easiest in threes: Eat, drink and be merry. Jesus told a lame man, "Arise, take up thy bed and walk."

And more: On your mark, get set, go!

Snap, crackle and pop.

Rub-a-dub-dub, three men in a tub.

I could get carried away with this. Like waltzing, the examples are endless and dizzying: one-two-three, one-two-three, one-two-three. So much more mesmerizing than the two-step.

Enough. The Engler triplets will see the magic of three all around them as they grow.

I wish them each a good dose of faith, hope and charity. A safe dose of sex, drugs and rock 'n' roll. And opportunities for health, wealth and happiness, every morning, noon and night.

November 15, 1994

All-American gluttony

We're getting fatter, all of us, adults and children, black and white. It's one slim thing we have in common as Americans. Everything separates us — race, gender, politics — except our fat.

We have no one to blame but ourselves, and American food purveyors who know we can't say no and offer us jumbo bags of potato chips and all-you-can-eat buffets.

Those buffets are deadly. They ought to be outlawed by Congress, out of concern for the public health. Nobody ought to be able to eat that way — three pounds of food for $4.95 — just as nobody ought to be able to ride a motorcycle without a helmet or receive a blood transfusion that hasn't been tested for HIV.

All-you-can-eat has now hit Japan. Men gorge on all-you-can-eat moo shu pork and women reportedly select up to 12 slices of cheesecake at an all-you-can-eat cheesecake emporium — $15 for whatever you can swallow.

We do not often see obese Japanese, except for those who earn their livings in sumo wrestling.

But we will. Japan will balloon as America and most of Western civilization has. Only Parisians and the very poor will remain thin.

I once spent most evenings in all-you-can-eat spots. I was a college student who, when I started, weighed 123 pounds. By the time I graduated four years later I weighed 147 and endured this endearment from my boyfriend: "chipmunk cheeks."

A previous boyfriend and I, both editors at the student newspaper, scheduled our meals around the all-you-can-eat specials common in East Lansing.

Our thinking was this: We worked sooo hard and sooo long today that we deserve a huuuge meal.

Food as reward. The more heroic we were on Wednesday, the more helpings of HoJo's fried clams we deserved.

Food as solace. The more unhappy we were on Sunday, the more unpleasant our chores, the more we deserved a third heaping plateful of spaghetti and a few extra slabs of garlic toast.

Eating to justify expense. Even now, an $8.95 breakfast buffet makes me nervous. Nothing tastes very good, but I'm paying $8.95, so I better try to eat my money's worth.

How stupid can we be?

I would still weigh 123 pounds if when I was young I had instead decided I deserved a small but very fine dinner: a two- or three-ounce cut of filet mignon, for example. Or a quarter-cupful of Russian caviar on toast. Or a small plate of exotic greens with wedges of homegrown beefsteak tomatoes, a shaving of imported provolone and a drizzle of extra-virgin, cold-pressed olive oil.

I didn't know then that most of the time you have to spend more to gain less.

For example: My local store sells 14-ounce bags of potato chips, on sale, for $1.99. A two-ounce bag costs 60 cents. You'd be a financial fool to choose the small bag over the large bag. Such a deal it is! And only 1,200 calories! Not that you will eat the whole thing, of course, unless you're deep in self-pity or TV.

Food purveyors ought to be required to make larger portions cost lots more. If a small bag of chips costs 60 cents, a bag twice as big should cost three times as much. If one plate of spaghetti is $2.95, the second plate should add an additional $5 to your bill, and the third an additional $8 on top of that.

Such restaurants might be called all-you-can-pay, forcing us to choose between our two great loves: calories or cash.

A tough call, but I think we'd make the right one.

October 12, 1995

The fine print

Because I was far from home, and needed news of the world, I went to a local supermarket to buy the Sunday New York Times.

"Geez," said the young clerk to me as she rang it up, $4.25. "It keeps getting more expensive, even though the paper it's on is probably worth only 25 cents."

Her comment struck me as curious. I said, "I don't buy it for its paper. I buy it for its intelligence."

The bagger wandered over. "Look at how small the type is!" he said. He screwed up his face in distaste. "That's what I look for first in a book — big type."

The clerk said, "I look for pictures. Without pictures, what's the point of reading? And they've got to be color pictures."

The bagger nodded. The clerk, feeling empowered, then said, "Actually, I don't read at all."

The bagger laughed. "I look for books that have been made into movies, and I think, 'Three hours reading or three hours watching?' You know what always wins."

I, meanwhile, tucked under my arm my newspaper with its tiny type and black-and-white pictures and walked to my car feeling blue. If two kids in a Midwestern city with exceptional schools don't care to read unless the type is big and the pictures are bright, what future is there for them? Or for we who deal in black type on white paper?

We believe mere words can travel to readers' minds like a laser beam, etching ideas and information, forcing open new frontiers in their imaginations.

As I left that supermarket, I felt foolish. I'm deluding myself, I thought. I'm like the shoe repairmen or seamstresses who tell themselves their work is important, while the rest of us throw away our old shoes and buy our clothes off the rack.

That evening, though, I went home with my brother and his wife and their two boys, 7 and 9. We adults read my newspaper, trading sections. My sister-in-law jotted in a notebook the names of books she wanted to check out the next day at the local Barnes & Noble, which her sons know by name and like to visit.

The boys were sent to bed without their usual permission to read, exhausted after a rough-and-tumble day. Typically, though, they are allowed to take flashlights to bed, and sometimes lie for an hour with their books, reading in an intimate glow that makes the darkness cozy.

"Why do you read books?" I asked my nephews. "To be a better reader," said Brian, who is 7. "And to learn stuff."

"The fantasy ones are good," said Chris, who is 9, "because you can imagine things, and maybe go into another world."

I asked if their friends read as much as they do. "Oh, they wanna play outside all the time, or watch TV," said Chris. Do their parents have anything to do with whether they read? Chris thought a minute. "No," he said. "Some kids just like to read, and some don't, and some don't know how."

But those of us older than 9 know where the credit and blame lie. Reading is an everyday thing in my nephews' home. On their kitchen refrigerator hang two yellow sheets of paper, each labeled "List of Books Read for Summer Reading Contract," a voluntary school program. Chris has already listed one book and Brian two, although vacation just started.

Me, I took to bed a dog-eared paperback called "The Castle in the Attic," by Elizabeth Winthrop, which Chris loaned to me, saying, "Aunt Susan, I really liked this book and I thought maybe you would like to read it in bed. If you don't finish it while you're here, you can take it home and give it back next time." What a thrilling offer, to share a book with my nephew — a wonderful omen of exciting worlds to come.

June 13, 1995

He's got avocado's number

In the grand scheme of things, an avocado is nothing — a fruit picked from a tree, peeled, eaten and forgotten.

Cutting it is here and gone, and not worth worrying over.

Which is why Mark Henning's way with an avocado is worth noting.

Mark is a line cook in an Ann Arbor restaurant frequented by students and faculty. He is paid $10.70 an hour. His work in the kitchen of the Red Hawk Bar & Grill is remarkable for only two reasons: He is impeccably neat, with an apron that stays white and clean throughout his eight-hour shift.

And he can cut an avocado into 75 slices, then fan them onto a plate like a deck of cards, and then some.

You think this is nothing? Then go out and buy an avocado and tell me, please, if you can cut it into anywhere near 75 slices.

I hit 28. Or 32, if I am very slow and careful and follow Mark's instructions. Maybe it's my knife. Maybe it's my avocado. Or maybe some of us are good at some things, and not so good at others.

Mark is 29, the son of a dietitian who taught all her children to cook, and a Goodyear draftsman who just retired after 40 years.

"I attribute a lot of what I am to my dad," Mark tells me when, in a booth at the Red Hawk, I ask him what compels him to do what he does to a simple avocado.

"My dad was very meticulous about the way he did everything and now, even if I wanted to do something halfway, I can't."

When co-owner Dick Schubach concocted the Red Hawk's menu, he put a dish called Southwestern Crab Cake with Avocado on it: "Snow and stone crab claw meat grilled with red and green chiles, scallions and red mole sauce." He wanted a sliced avocado alongside the crab cake, to brighten it.

"I took it as a personal challenge," Mark told me, "to see how many slices I could get." Just as, I found out, he took it as a challenge to pay his own way through U-M, "without any handouts from my parents." He is a semester away, after 10 years of effort, from earning a bachelor's degree in computer-aided design and manufacturing.

After Mark hit the mid-70s in avocado slices, Red Hawk cooks competed to top him.

No one has, and no one even tries anymore.

Says Schubach: "It's very heartening to see someone go out of their way to do more than we ask them to do."

Mark showed me his trick in the Red Hawk kitchen last week, only slightly sheepish while his fellow cooks looked on and teased him.

He halved an avocado lengthwise, pitted it, peeled one half, and set it west to east in front of him on a cutting board. Instead of slicing it right to left, as any right-handed person would slice a loaf of bread, he cut from the left. He cupped his left hand over the knife to hold the avocado in place, pressing his left thumb gently so the slices he just made wouldn't ride up on the knife.

It helps, Mark said, to have a nicely ripe avocado — not too mushy, not too hard — and a very sharp, very wide knife.

Finally, he fanned the slices by nudging them with the flat of the knife, pushing away from himself.

Maybe you had to be there.

Mark admitted last week that I was the only diner to ever compliment his avocado, which he has sliced in the same way for hundreds of crab cake plates.

"I don't get much feedback," he told me.

Nobody gets much feedback — one reason why so many people don't bother doing any more than they must. But it can't be the only reason, because Mark keeps slicing his avocados the best he can.

August 25, 1995

Congratulations, graduates

Let us commence this season of commencement speeches by bearing in mind one essential truth:

People don't like wisdom shoved down their throats.

Yet people famous and obscure will continue to try to do it, the way parents shove mittens in their children's coat pockets as the kids rush out the door.

Wisdom tastes like pea soup when you're 22 and somebody is standing at a lectern spoon-feeding it to you.

It's much better when you discover it for yourself, sometime later, often when you're in crisis.

But, in any case, long after the graduation party is over.

Some big-time universities actually pay commencement speakers as much as $15,000.

Graduating students can imagine better ways to spend such big money, but it's spent for the benefit of parents, who do listen to commencement speakers and nod in happy agreement.

Parents are particularly impressed when a university to which they've paid an amount approaching the gross national product of some Third World country hires someone "big" to speak. Someone like, say, Tom Hanks.

Here are commencement speakers' favorite themes:

■ Dream the impossible dream.

■ Ask not what your country can do for you, but what you can do for your country.

■ To thine own self be true.

■ Challenge authority.

■ Keep your chin up.

■ Money isn't everything.

Yep. Sure. Yawn.

What my stepson remembers best about his commencement speaker at Eastern Michigan University is that while she droned on, he and his pals enjoyed a bottle of champagne he managed to sneak in beneath his gown.

In many ways commencement speeches are a lot like wedding sermons.

A minister's words about love and marriage bring tears to the eyes of nearly everybody in the church: the long-marrieds, the once- (or twice- or thrice-) marrieds, the not-yet-marrieds.

But the bride and groom, they've got other things on their minds.

I couldn't find anyone who remembered a single remark from his or her commencement speaker. This doesn't mean all those words fell on deaf (or drunken) ears.

Little droplets of wisdom do plop on our heads and sink into our brains now and again. We tend to forget where we were, though, when insight struck. We might well have been in an auditorium.

Somehow we all learned that every gray cloud has a silver lining. That success is 1 percent inspiration and 99 percent perspiration. And that if some awful thing doesn't kill you, it will make you stronger.

As a nation, we Americans don't ask a lot of wisdom. It needn't be deep as long as it's catchy. Witness "Life is like a box of chocolates: You never know what you're going to get."

Duh.

Therefore, in closing, I suggest scrapping all commencement speeches and allowing graduates to issue advice to each other — in five words or less.

Hand them their diplomas, then let them step to the mike and let their words fly. Some may squander their opportunity with something self-serving like "Go Wings!"

But you can say a lot that's important in five words or less:

Seize the day. Live and let live. Let's love one another.

And: My time is now up.

May 30, 1996